Introduction to

HEALTH FOODS

By Marjorie Miller

NASH PUBLISHING
LOS ANGELES

CONTENTS

RECIPES

WHY HEALTH FOODS?

People began to leave their farms and move into cities about a hundred years ago. The devitalization of foods began then—with the improper milling of wheat.

The germ of the grain was removed and discarded for practical reasons of storage, from motives of profit, and to satisfy people's ideas of what was elegant. The nutritious whole-grain loaf, associated with country people, was gradually replaced by the refined, white loaf, associated with wealth.

The nutrients of the grain, contained in the germ, were fed to cattle and pigs who grew healthy on it. The starch of the grain, contained in the remainder of the wheat kernel, was fed to people who grew ill from it.

Within fifty years, national health had declined significantly. By the Second World War, so many American men were unfit for military service, so many civilians lacked good health, that a national program of "enrichment" for white bread was begun. Vitamins—made synthetically—were put back into the white loaf and people relaxed. At least some people did. Others were curious. If synthetic vitamins

11

were being added for health, where were those that they were replacing. They were found—in feeding troughs and bins.

A "health food" was born—the wheat germ itself, wheat germ oil, and the bran of the wheat germ.

Scientists, busy in their laboratories, continued to experiment with synthetics.

Nutritionists continued to look for missing nutrients and found them—in blackstrap molasses, the residue of refined white sugar. While valuable stock animals were winning blue ribbons for health, *people* were eating refined sugar and visiting their dentists.

They found nutrients in foods that were new to this country but had been used in other cultures for centuries—yogurt, a tart, custardlike food with legends of Bulgarians who ate it and lived to a hundred years and beyond.

Nutritionists found them in *seeds*—exotic, foreign seeds like the sesame. Seeds native to the American Indian—like the sunflower.

The soybean—the lowly soybean—was found to contain an astonishing number of health-giving values. Not so astonishing to the millions of Orientals whose staple diet it had been for centuries.

Herbs were rediscovered. In some kitchens they had never been lost, but the medicinal and health-giving properties of herbs, known since the Middle Ages and earlier, were viewed with renewed interest.

The nutritionists knew what they were looking for.

The discovery of vitamins at the turn of the century had provided one of the keys to the puzzle.

Dutch and English scientists had discovered that an absence of something in a food could cause disease. Further experiments proved *that there were forty nutrients essential to good health.* Further, that preferably these forty should be supplied in foods at the same time.

A Dr. Weston Price set out to find some healthy people and to study what they ate. He found them among groups that lived close to the land, in various parts of the world; people who for one reason or another had not been affected by civilization.

He found them in the Swiss Alps and in northern Italy. In Australia, New Zealand, Central America, the South American jungles, and in the far north of Canada and Alaska.

What were these people like? They stood straight and tall, they had much physical endurance, they had good dispositions. Their teeth had stayed free from decay and their bodies free from disease. There was no evidence of any of the diseases modern man suffers from.

What were they eating? What did their diets have in common? Were they all eating yogurt? Or drinking goat's milk? Or eating whole-grain foods to the exclusion of animal foods?

Some were. Some weren't.

Some ate meat and fish almost exclusively.

Some ate vegetables and grains.

But their diets had two things in common. Whatever they ate, investigation showed that *their foods met every body requirement*--even though the source of calcium, for example, might be from ground whalebone in one instance and lime from dishes used in grinding corn in another.

Second, or perhaps first, they did not know how to refine foods. They ate them in their natural state.

Three hundred years ago, the early settlers of this country lived in a similar way. All the food was grown on the healthy virgin soil of young America. We associate strength and endurance with those early pioneers.

The growing population of the country, and with it, mass production, brought the use of chemical fertilizers on the soil, the invention of machinery for milling grains, new ways of forcing hybrid crops to yield higher tonnage per acre on worn-out soil, and new methods of refining and processing foods.

We have become one of the most overfed, undernourished nations in history. Today, of the eight thousand products on the shelves of our supermarkets, over five thousand have been "invented" by biochemists since World War II. Synthetic flavorings, synthetic foods such as eggs and nuts, synthetic colorings.

Young people in America are rebelling. Critical of the synthetics which have become a part of the American way of living, they are popularizing what has been a steadily growing movement by nutritionists to combat the harm done by the increasing deluge of processed, refined, empty foods.

They are advocating a return to natural living, to food grown as the pioneers in this country grew it. That's what "granny" glasses are saying—that's what long calico skirts and bare feet are all about—young people nostaligic, as well as resentful of the technological, computerized age we're living in.

And they're doing something about it. Many of them have "taken to the hills" to do their own organic gardening, bake their own fresh, nutritious, whole-grain breads.

On campuses throughout the country, students are working in their own organic flower and vegetable gardens. They're spreading mulch and compost materials—using no chemical fertilizers. In their college dining halls they're eating corn on the cob just off the stalk, ripe tomatoes, and fresh string beans that they have grown themselves.

They're working in food stores. They call themselves *organic merchants*. These stores have a special atmosphere of their own, reflecting interests in Oriental religions, folk music, and the old-fashioned country store, with big crocks of sesame seed oil and soy sauce, barrels and tins of bulk grains and seeds.

The foods in a health food store, selected by organic merchants, have been bought for their nutritional value. And they taste good.

"We're not," these merchants say, "interested in selling you perfect-looking foods. Our apples aren't all exactly the same size with the same tint of redness. But each isn't more tasteless than the last.

"Our organically grown fruits and vegetables haven't been waxed and they haven't been dyed to make you think they're fresher or more colorful than they really are.

"In a health food store you can buy any kind of grain or cereal product you can think of—and probably quite a few you may not have realized existed. *Whole*-grain flour and *whole*-grain cereals—without preservatives or chemicals.

"We have brown rice or wild rice. Breakfast cereals: hot, cold, quick-cooking, or the kind that take longer to cook.

"You can buy bread mixes, pancake mixes, wheat germ, rice polish, rice flour, rye flour and millet—a very tasty and nourishing cereal food.

"And we have bread already baked. The bakers we buy from are interested in one thing—nourishing you. You can find rye bread, whole-wheat bread, cracked-wheat bread, wheat germ bread, or bread made from a number of mixed flours. There's also a flourless loaf—made chiefly from whole-grain berries that have been sprouted for greater nutritional value.

"Honey—that amazing product of an equally amazing creature, the bee—is available in almost limitless varieties. You can buy the dark kind, like buckwheat, which contains more vitamins and minerals than the light kind and is generally only available in health food stores.

"You may buy honey in the comb or in the liquid form. And honey that is guaranteed to be as free from pesticides as it is humanly possible to make. These bees haven't been fed sugar and water during the winter, as some commercially owned bees are.

"Drinking too much coffee? Try herb teas—like grandmother used to make. You'll find every flavor available—herb, flower, or leaf teas. Drink them for pleasure and good health. Or try coffee substitutes made from grains or soybeans.

"If you're trying to eat less salt, you'll find herbs, seaweeds, and other harmless foods as substitutes.

"And if chocolate is making you fat, try carob. It's an interesting, satisfying food.

"We have protein supplements for extra energy—pills, wafers, cookies, crackers, powder, or liquid—anything that suits you.

"Seed foods—they're great as snacks and full of protein and vitamins and minerals. Nuts—exotic, tropical nuts high in proteins and nutritious oils. The soybean—in all its forms.

"We also carry many canned fruits and vegetables, also frozen foods, along with our fresh, raw vegetables and fruit juices. All of these have been organically grown.

"Our dairy products include foods you probably can't buy anywhere else: goat's milk, goat's cheese, raw, certified milk, yogurt in many different flavors, yogurt makers and 'starters,' and cheeses—hard, soft, with or without mold."

Health food stores also carry vitamin and mineral supplements in combinations or as individual vitamins and minerals. Organic merchants buy natural food supplements—which means that the vitamins and minerals in the product have been derived from a natural food, such as yeast or kelp. The food supplement also contains a small amount of the nutritious food itself, which is good since there may be other undiscovered elements in the food which are important, too. In a natural-food supplement there will be many that are still unknown, because, of course, they all exist in natural foods.

Dr. Weston Price didn't report the use of food supplements in the Swiss Alps or the Arctic. But neither did those places have air pollution or water pollution or crowded cities or chemicals in foods to contend with.

SLOW POISON

Meats and dairy products today are full of chemicals, drugs, hormones, and preservatives. All of them unknown a hundred years ago.

Cereals are refined to the point where they can hardly be called a cereal. Fresh fruits and vegetables, which are no longer seasonal but available the year around, are contaminated with insecticides, preservatives, waxes, dyes, and hundreds of other chemicals that were unknown in earlier times.

Many fats have been denatured—treated with bleaches and hydrogenated. The original fatty acids are changed into entirely different chemical compounds. Modern food is convenient, but the *quality* of its nourishment has decreased, while the content of its chemicals has increased.

We are eating an impressive array of chemicals and synthetic foods, but the figures for heart disease and cancer are steadily increasing. Tests indicate that at least some of these chemicals may be cancer causing. Processed fats and refined sugar have been shown to have a relation to heart and blood vessel disease.

There are over a thousand chemicals being used in foods. They're being added in two ways—one not intentional. Poisons are absorbed into food from insecticides, fumicides, and weed-killers.

It is a fallacy to believe that chemical sprays are necessary. With proper farming methods they are not. Healthy soils produce fruits and vegetables that are immune to most fungus diseases and insects.

DDT is highly toxic. There is also no known antidote. It is absorbed by plants and cannot be removed. It is also absorbed by humans who eat those plants.

Milk is especially affected by it. DDT is fat-soluble and has been found in milk from cows whose only contact with it was through sprays used in dairies. Animals fed on hay that has been sprayed with it are also affected.

When fruit trees are sprayed with DDT or other poisonous insecticides—and they are sometimes sprayed eight times during a growing season—not only are the fruits contaminated, but spray falls on the ground. Plants grown in that soil receive a concentrated dosage.

We may be eating antibiotics and hormones we weren't intending to eat. In one instance, farmers were unable to make cheese because one cow, treated with penicillin, had absorbed the chemical, and the organisms for cheese making in the whole batch of milk were destroyed.

Are we unsuspectingly being dosed with antibiotics?

Are we also getting hormones we don't intend to take?

The practice of feeding animals with synthetic hormones raises questions which, as yet, have not been answered. The hormones fill the fat tissues of the animal with water. Their weight is increased. We buy meat by the pound. What do the hormones do to us? Do they have an effect on water retention in our bodies? What of high protein reducing diets? What of the trend toward "unisex" fashions. Implausible?

Perhaps. Impossible? It's difficult to say with certainty.

Chemicals are also put into our foods. The purpose being either to change the food itself or to preserve it beyond its natural life.

The food is then both artificial *and* stale.

There are over one thousand chemicals that take the place of eggs, fats, and other nutrients.

There are some five hundred synthetic flavorings which manufacturers are allowed to use in place of fruit or nuts or herbs. The taste is there—the nutrients are not.

Natural fruit extracts—the oils of oranges or lemons—are more expensive than synthetic extracts. They can be produced under controllable conditions. Mass produced. Some foods do contain natural flavorings—banana oil, vanilla extract. We also eat some unnatural ones—amyl acetate, benzaldehyde, carvone, ethyl butyrate, and methyl salicylate.

We eat chemicals that have been added to keep foods from caking. Have you noticed that your brown sugar doesn't turn hard as a rock if the weather happens to have been damp? Salt pours freely and cake mixes don't get hard. If you had your choice, would you rather have to pulverize the brown sugar or as a "side dish" eat some calcium aluminum silicate, magnesium carbonate, or perhaps a pinch of sodium aluminum silicate? If you shop in a supermarket, you don't even have the choice.

The pasteboard personality, so identified with modern society, is as much a result of things we don't have to do for ourselves anymore as it is of our emptiness in other areas.

At first, "convenience" was like a glittering bauble on a Christmas tree. People were glad to be freed of those little annoyances when they had so many more important things to do.

In the 1950s, the era of "convenience foods" was born. These were busy, affluent years. Mass communication was in'creased through television to an extent not known before. Commercials supported the new medium; the consumer was its target. Advertising set the trends.

Women were more and more a part of the business world—their needs changed. No longer at home during the day to prepare meals, the TV dinner was welcomed. The TV dinner. The instant pudding. The ready-whip whip cream.

In the last twenty years, the deluge has increased. So have crime, poor health, and anxiety. People were being freed to be happier, more productive. Is it unreasonable to suggest that we are caught in a cycle—that our personalities, in part, reflect what we're eating? The man being slowly poisoned by minute quantities of lead arsenate doesn't know it. The best detective writers and readers know that. He just doesn't feel quite well.

There are residues of lead arsenates on our fruits, on our vegetables, and in our salads.

By the time those fruits have been made into jellies and preserves, there are residues of other things, too. There are antifoaming agents—one in particular called dimethylpolysiloxane. Harmful? The Pure Food and Drug Commission says not. They didn't think cyclamates were, either.

The nature of bread is changed by a bleaching agent. People wanted their bread bleached. The manufacturer is not entirely to blame. He must please the consumer. If people wanted fluffy, snowy white loaves, then he obliged by figuring out a way to give them what they wanted. "White" bread was associated with elegance, and from a practical point of view, it was evidence that there were no impurities in the bread. Who prefers bits of bugs and dirt?

White bread was also a status symbol. So bread manufacturers found ways to bleach flour.

The first bleach used, in England, was found to be highly

toxic and was removed from the market. Others have replaced it.

By using a bleach, manufacturers discovered that they could sell inferior grades of flour.

Flour should bleach naturally. This takes months. It's making no one a profit while the aging process occurs. It's also a nuisance to store. To process it quickly makes money and is convenient. Never mind that it's not as healthful.

High quality grades of wheat were artificially oxidized and lightened. It was also discovered that inferior grades of wheat, which would never bleach naturally to a high quality, could be made to seem so if artificially bleached.

When you buy a loaf of bread today, read the label. You may pay a little more for unbleached flour as an ingredient, but you're getting a much higher grade of bread—more nutritious as well as free of the bleaching agent. One less chemical you've eaten for breakfast, or lunch, or dinner.

Chemicals are added as *emulsifying agents* to keep fatty particles in suspension in liquids. You might have to stir up the jar of mayonnaise or peanut butter, and that's a nuisance, but would you rather be eating propylene glycol alginate?

Or how about some shellac? Or beeswax? Or any of the other various substances that are added to foods when a nice glaze is needed. There are other ways of making glazes—with natural wholesome ingredients. But they cost more. You'll buy the product, probably, that tastes the best and costs the least. We've been educated that way. Our Puritan forefathers liked economy—Madison Avenue dreamed up the glamour. It's glamorous to be slender, too. Men are considered more handsome that way. And what are the best women? Thin and rich, of course.

When the body is starved of nutrients, the blood-sugar level drops. What are you hungry for? Sugar. A delicious slice of chocolate layer cake, a rich, creamy sundae, a piece of pie.

What your body really needs is some nourishing food. But it doesn't know that anymore. We've lost the ability to discriminate between taste and nourishment. We wouldn't eat sixteen apples, but we eat that much sugar in a candy bar. We know we shouldn't eat the sugar, but we want it. Manufacturers and biochemists have obligingly invented sugar substitutes.

We've been eating and drinking cyclamates for twenty years. They are derived from a substance once used to clean out boilers. They have been removed from the market. They may cause cancer.

We've been using saccharin for quite a while, too. It's four hundred times as sweet as sugar. It's a white crystalline compound made from coal tar.

Salt was man's first preservative and his main preservative for centuries. He has recently invented hundreds more. Antioxidants help preserve the freshness of foods by combating rancidity of oils and fats. Such chemicals as propyl gallate and butylated hydroxyanisole are used in cheeses and other foods which may grow rancid if kept too long.

We eat chemicals of the nitrate group in meats such as weiners. Nitrates preserve color and freshness. Nitrates from the soil, absorbed into plants have been shown to be poisonous.

Antistaling agents are put into cakes and breads. This means that bakery goods can be kept longer by the manufacturer and by the seller before they reach us.

It has not been proved that the loaf of bread hasn't deteriorated. Just that it doesn't seem stale. You may start your day with a preservative. In your glass of juice you may also drink a little benzoic acid. In your glass of milk, hydrogen peroxide. Or perhaps some oat gum. Or perhaps both.

Have you wondered why ice cream doesn't taste as good anymore? Here's what else you may be eating: an emulsifier, a thickening agent, a neutralizer, a buffer, some artificial flavoring, a bactericide, and an antioxicant. That means some more oat gum, some agar-agar, some mono- and di-glycerides, some calcium carbonate, some hydrogen peroxide.

Cottage cheese gives you a nice variety of chemicals, too: annatto, which is a vegetable dye, cochineal, which is another dye and is made from the dried bodies of a tropical American insect, and diacetyl, which is a butter flavoring.

We are, indeed, eating an impressive array of chemicals and synthetic foods.

As someone remarked, however, when man starts competing with nature in the blending of food elements, it would be well for him to be sure that his formula does not bear the mark of the medicine cabinet—the skull and the crossbones.

NATURE'S NOURISHMENT

Mountain climbing is a vigorous sport. Sir Edmund Hillary carried honey with him when he scaled Mt. Everest. He was eating one of the oldest foods known to man.

Scientists know the exact chemical composition of honey. It contains three types of sugar, vitamins, and minerals. A small amount of protein.

But scientists can't make honey in a laboratory. There is some substance, occurring in the natural product, that cannot be reproduced.

Nature seems to be the best judge of what will keep us in good health. The seed is an excellent example.

Perhaps the most balanced, consistent combination of health-giving nutrients is found in the seed. Research has shown that nature has protected its source of life.

An experiment with chemical fertilizers showed that a highly concentrated dose of phosphorus was absorbed into the leaves of the plant, but the seed was not affected.

In some way that we don't understand, the seed is able to protect itself against harmful substances. The seed absorbs from the soil what it needs to sustain itself and the life of the plant. It cannot, however, absorb minerals from the soil that are not there.

In a psychedelic bookstore in Los Angeles, there's a showcase of cards. One of them has this quote with the accompanying comment:

> And God said, Behold, I have given you every herb bearing seed, which is upon the face of the earth, and every tree, in which is the fruit of a tree yielding seed; to you it shall be for meat.
>
> —Gen. 1:29
> *Subject to a higher authority*

Young people are feeling that the "establishment" has tried to play God.

Man lived for literally millions of years on this earth, eating what nature would yield. Before he settled down, he roamed the earth—looking for food. Before there was any agriculture—before recorded history—man lived in the tropics and ate fruits, berries, and roots—he was a "gatherer."

Later, when he moved farther north, he became a hunter and a herdsman, living on foods from animals—meat and milk—and any of his former vegetables that he could still find. Large communities weren't possible—there was never that much food in one place.

It is possible to say that the discovery of the cultivation of cereal marked the beginning of civilization. Man found that there were certain grasses he could plant and harvest. Food could be stored and eaten in the winter. A permanent home could be established under these conditions; he didn't have to move when the seasons changed or when game disappeared.

Early civilizations developed where food was plentiful. The ancient Egyptians could and did grow three crops a year on the rich soils of the Nile River Basin. The climate was warm—they raised fruits and vegetables and grains. Beans and peas, melons, grapes—and wheat. Basic foods. Nutritious foods.

The Egyptians baked bread. They had wild game and fish. They roasted antelopes and ducks, pigeons and sheep over charcoal fires. The extra food they preserved by pickling or smoking or salting. They used no chemical fertilizers on their soil. No artificial coloring on their fruits.

The Hebrews lived more simply. They had so much milk from domestic goats and so much honey from wild bees that their home lands became known as the Land of Milk and Honey.

Goat's milk has a distinctive flavor and is highly nutritious; honey is considered one of nature's most health-giving foods.

The Hebrews also ate rice and wheat and barley. They baked bean-flour bread and made a thick, lentil soup called pottage.

The early Greeks and Romans were the first to reach out into other countries for food. Figs and grapes were native to their countries. They raised domestic animals, ate seafoods, and used wheat and barley for bread and porridge. They "buttered" their bread with olive oil; their grapes they fermented to make wine.

In Iran they found cherries.

In the Orient, apricots, peaches and spices.

In Africa, fish.

From Egypt they brought back other grains, and from Syria, plums and dates. They raised fish in ponds. And they were the first to set out oyster beds.

After the Roman Empire fell in the fifth century, Europe could no longer trade with other countries. Feudal lords couldn't import goods; they depended on their own resources for food. People grew grain and vegetables but they had little to feed either themselves or their animals.

But between the years 1000 and 1300, trade was resumed between Europe and the East. The Crusades took place. As a result, new foods were eaten and new tastes were acquired. When these Europeans returned home, their desire for better food helped renew trade and influenced the exploration of new lands.

Man's need to eat—to nourish himself—has influenced civilization continuously.

Columbus found America, and proved that the world wasn't flat, but it was *spices* for which he was looking.

He didn't find any spices, but he did find some new vegetables. Corn and sweet and white potatoes were unknown to Europe until the sixteenth century.

Spanish explorers in South America brought back to Europe with them the cassava roots, from which tapioca is made and cacao beans, the bean that we make chocolate with.

The early American colonists ate most of these foods. They had large quantities of fish, game, nuts, and wild fruits. Colonial farmers grew beans and corn and pumpkins—a vegetable underrated today but nutritious—and other vegetables. They raised pigs and sheep and cattle.

The American Indians showed them where to find salt, and using it as a preservative, they had food in winter. They smoked hams, cured meats, and salted fish.

We're hopefully going back to a healthier way of living. Astrologists call it the Age of Aquarius—the age of humanity. Eric Fromm calls it a "Revolution of Hope. Toward a Humanized Technology."

Today we have available to us some, if not all, of those foods known to man for centuries. We are able to evaluate them now and understand and appreciate their health-giving properties. Many "health foods" consist of foods like the soybean, which we realize now contains an abundance of nutrients. We are gaining new respect for wheat and other whole grains, the staple of much of the western world. Fruits and vegetables and nuts have been analyzed for their nutritious value, and we are gaining new understanding of their importance. What we once considered an inferior diet based on nonmeat products, we are finding has sustained health for people when the necessary balance of nutrients was present.

There is still a question about the health-giving values of meat and meat products. It is possible, although it takes planning and knowledge of nutrition, to be a well-nourished vegetarian. Most nutritionists in this country, however, feel that meat and meat products are essential for optimum health. We are fortunate that we are free to choose. As we are also free to choose between synthetic and natural foods.

We are a wealthy, industrial economy. We can afford meats, which are expensive. We can afford to import food from other countries—any of the nutritious foods which we don't grow here.

It is ironic that while we are becoming well-aware of the need for high protein foods, we are being sold and are eating junk in this country. A large manufacturer of synthetic foods, for American markets, also manufacturers a protein supplement which is sent to undernourished countries. Charity ought to begin at home.

We are having to enrich our diet with the soybean, while we send protein supplements abroad.

If man hadn't devised machinery which removed the germ of grain from the kernel, we probably would be having fewer health problems in this country. A hundred years ago, we ate a lot of whole-grain foods and with them a good supply of B vitamins, vitamin E, unsaturated fatty acids, and other nutrients. It is estimated that the average intake of vitamin E at the turn of the century was 150 grams daily. Today, in an average diet, we get 7 grams or so.

But we are hopefully gaining a greater appreciation for food, a greater respect for those foods which, in a predominantly meat-eating country, we have gradually gotten away from—and, an understanding of what a diet high in refined sugars and low in nutritional values may be doing to our health.

In the panorama of man's history, grain has played a significant part. It was responsible for communal living, for what we understand as civilization. It is easy to forget that there have been highly evolved civilizations and ones that have been less so. Our culture is frequently compared to the Roman Empire, which fell from decadence within.

The Bible calls bread the staff of life. Bread is made from grains. For centuries it has been the largest single food item used throughout the world. The refining process, invented only within the last one hundred years, has produced an empty food. Studies have shown that what the cereal grain contains, in varying quantities, is vitamin E—now thought to be essential for vigor and fertility.

It might be said that much of the national health of a country depends on the quality of its bread. Almost everyone in the world eats bread of some kind. Whether it is sweet or sour, brown or white, heavy or light, it is made from flour. And all flour comes from grain.

From the seeds of such plants as wheat, rice, rye, and oats, we also get cooked rice, cooked oats, cooked corn, and other cooked grain. If we devitalize these grains, we only short-change ourselves. The choice is ours.

We either import or grow in this country most of the fruits and vegetables or variations of them that men have eaten for centuries. Many of ours are becoming tasteless. They are grown on worn-out soils, picked before they are ripe, colored, waxed, and otherwise made unpalatable and unnutritious. But there are a wide variety of potentially nutritious foods available to us. "Health foods" are not just alfalfa sprouts and desiccated liver, although you may find either or both to your taste and certainly both are nutritious. But we're becoming acquainted again with fruits and vegetables—the garden variety and the more exotic ones.

Of the foods that we have come to call fruits and vegetables, we eat various parts—some more susceptible to poisonous sprays than others.

We eat the roots of beets, carrots, and sweet potatoes; we eat the leaves of cabbage, lettuce, and spinach. At least we might like to. Some sprays that are used on lettuce are so oily that they can't be washed off. We eat the stems of the nutritious asparagus and the stalks of celery. Celery, which is rich in chlorophyll, is frequently bleached with a gas process to produce a whiter stalk that people seem to find more attractive.

We eat the bulbs of onions and the flours of cauliflower and broccoli.

Cucumbers, peppers, and tomatoes are really the fruits of plants. Botanists say we're eating vegetables, or vegetable-fruits, if you like. Trees are also considered plants, and their fruits are usually classified as fruits. Apples, berries, figs, lemons, olives, and oranges—rich with natural sugars and juices—or they should be.

Spices come from other parts of plants. The clove is the dried flower bud of a tropical evergreen. We buy cloves in the store—do we think about how they grow in their natural state? If we don't know what their natural state is, it's hard to judge how much they've been tampered with. The leaves of tea are, of course, from an evergreen plant grown in China and India. How much do we know of the many varieties of teas made from herbs? It used to be that herb gardens were common and their use widespread.

Meats and other animal products form a large part of the average American diet. It's estimated they make up some 30 to 40 percent of our total food intake. In countries like Ceylon, India, and South Africa, the food from animals may be less than 20 percent of the diet.

Protein, the main substance in the human body, is also the main substance in animal foods. Most nutritionists feel that animal proteins are more complete proteins than those found in vegetables.

In this country, we have available to us, the flesh of such animals as cattle, hogs, sheep, and poultry. Also, and highly nutritious, are internal organs such as hearts, kidneys, and livers. Liver has come to be grouped with the "wonder foods"—wheat germ, yogurt, brewer's yeast, and liver. This is because liver is extremely rich in vitamins, particularly the B vitamins and is one of the few sources of vitamin B_{12} .

We have fish available to us—a rich potential source of iodine and other valuable minerals and vitamins. In the days before pollution, healthy fish were found in clear mountain lakes and streams. Now their use is questioned by some nutritionists.

Ocean fish and sea food have been thought to be free of contamination until rather recently. Now, DDT has been found in ocean fish in Southern California, and Jacques Cousteau in a recent *Time* magazine article expressed concern for damage being done to this huge, unplanted food crop. There are, in this part of the world, commercial fishing areas along the entire Atlantic and Pacific Coasts, and the Gulf of Mexico, extending hundreds of miles out to sea. How extensive is the contamination?

Health food stores are beginning to carry meats and poultry for those who wish to include them in their diets. These meats come from animals that have been raised on organic feed under humane conditions. Bacon, ham, pork, and sausage from hogs nutritionally fed are rather high in calories but are good sources of proteins and contain vitamins and minerals. Lamb is a lower caloric meat and a good source of minerals such as calcium, phosphorus, and iron. From cattle, of course, we get a wide variety of cuts of meat. From the great cattle-raising states of this country, beef is shipped to all parts of the world. How much of the meat is full of hormones? Not beef that you buy in a health food store.

Chicken and turkey are important in the American diet. There is much questioning of the methods being used in raising poultry. Questions are asked which have yet to be answered about the effect of chaining chickens to pens for their natural lives and feeding them various chemicals to increase their weight or their egg production.

Health food stores carry fertilized eggs. Eggs are eaten frequently by most Americans. Unfortunately, some of the eggs that we eat have a nice yellow color, which isn't natural, and are unfertilized, which isn't natural either. Fertilized eggs simply mean that in the barnyard there was a rooster around.

And what of the milk we drink? How nutritious is it? Milk, cream, cheese, buttermilk—all of these contain valuable proteins and should be rich in vitamins and minerals. Milk is sent to dairy plants where other products are produced—butter, cream, cheese, buttermilk. These plants also produce the canned milk, the powdered milk, and the skimmed milk we buy. It is up to us to choose between pasteurized products, which many nutritionists feel contain few if any nutrients, and products made from raw certified milk and its products. Raw certified milk is subject to stringent regulations which were first devised some sixty years ago by an American physician.

We are drinking more goat's milk, a highly nutritious food with a distinctive flavor. To a school child, milk used to mean cow's milk. In southern Europe and the Middle East, the goat is "the poor man's cow." We seem to be finding that the rough brown bread of the peasant, and the honey that he ate, and the goat's milk that he drank, made him healthy.

In India they drink buffalo milk; in Lapland it's reindeer milk; in Tibet, milk from the Yak; and in Arabia milk from camels. These could all probably be considered "health foods," too, if the reindeer haven't been munching DDT, or the camels penicillin.

PRINCIPLES
OF GOOD NUTRITION

What should we be eating for good health?

There is no such thing as a "normal" diet. There are some rules for good nutrition, however, which, if understood and followed, enable us to eat what we're hungry for and also what we need for optimum health. Once these rules are understood, it becomes apparent why nutritionists have expressed so much concern over the average American diet. Even those trying to eat nourishing, well-balanced meals may not be getting the nutrients they need for health.

Cooking destroys vitamins and minerals; so does excessive exposure to air. Some vitamins and minerals are not utilized in the body unless others are present. Some foods give us many of the forty nutrients we need. Others only a few or none at all. Even though people differ in their nutritional needs, everyone needs to eat a diet in which the forty nutrients are amply furnished.

In a discussion of nutrition, it's usual to classify foods as protein, carbohydrate, or fat, and there is general agreement that we need some of each in our meals.

Foods have three main uses in the body. They provide materials for building and repair, for energy, and for digestion. The *building* and *repair* materials are proteins. The word protein comes from the Greek, meaning "of first importance." It is considered exactly that today. It's the main substance of all living tissue. Nails, hair, skin, muscles are all made of protein. If your muscles are sagging, you're not eating enough of this essential substance.

When you eat enough protein, you should have more *energy*. All energy is produced by means of enzymes. These are organic substances whose principal component is protein. Vitamins form part of certain enzymes. If you're eating inadequate protein, however, your body isn't able to form sufficient quantities of enzymes. Fatigue is the result.

Digestion is likely to suffer if your protein intake is inadequate. There are several reasons. The body doesn't manufacture enough enzymes—food isn't properly changed into smaller particles which can be absorbed by the body. The intestinal and stomach supports are muscular, and will get flabby without enough protein, and thus the proper mixing of digestive juices and enzymes with foods doesn't happen. It is generally known that weak intestinal muscles can be a factor in constipation.

If you're feeling waterlogged and think you need to reduce, you'll probably go on a high protein diet and may lose as much as ten pounds the first week. The reason is not necessarily that protein burned up the fat, as is so commonly supposed. Albumin is the key. Albumin is a protein which is produced by the liver when the body is being furnished the necessary nutrients in the diet. In a rather complicated process, albumin collects urine from the system. If the diet is so inadequate that enough albumin can't be formed, then waste materials aren't completely removed from the tissues and you may think you've gained weight.

Proteins

How much protein should we eat during the day? What are good sources of protein? What's the difference between animal and vegetable proteins?

Meat, fish, and fowl are excellent sources of complete protein. Their bodies are made up largely of proteins, too. One-fourth of a pound, which is an average serving, will give you from 14 to 22 grams of complete proteins. The fatter the meat, or the more bony, the fewer proteins. A serving of spareribs or link sausages or the bony parts of chicken will average from 10 to 15 grams. Liver, rump roast, breast of chicken will average from 18 to 22 grams. Hamburger, steaks, ham or pork chops, lobster, crab or fresh shrimp contain between 15 to 18 grams of protein.

Milk, buttermilk, powdered milk, and yogurt are also excellent sources. One quart of milk, either whole or skim, or a quart of buttermilk, contains 32 to 35 grams of complete protein.

Eggs and cheese contain proteins that are complete. One egg contains 6 grams; cheese varies according to the type. Two slices of Swiss cheese will give you from 10 to 12 grams.

Soybeans are a rich source of complete proteins; one-half cup of cooked soybeans contains 20 grams.

Brewer's yeast, which differs from baking yeast, is a rich, inexpensive source of complete proteins. One-half cup contains 50 grams of protein. Adelle Davis' famous Tiger's Milk Recipe uses brewer's yeast.

Nuts are sources of proteins; some contain complete proteins, others are incomplete.

Peas and beans, in the vegetable family, contain proteins, although they are not considered complete. If they are eaten as the only source of protein, there are certain nutrients which will be lacking.

Grains also contain proteins, considered complete unless the germ has been removed.

Proteins are made of amino acids. These are a group of nitrogenous organic compounds which are essential to metabolism.

We know of the existence of twenty-two of these. It's a little like the alphabet, though. Just as with the twenty-six letters in the alphabet, we can make thousands of words, in the same way many proteins can be made from different combinations of the amino acids.

Different parts of the body are composed of different combinations of the amino acids; different foods contain different combinations of them.

Digestion breaks proteins down into these acids and then the body utilizes what it needs.

Of the twenty-two amino acids, there are eight which the body can manufacture. These have come to be referred to as the essential eight, although that's a little misleading since all of the others are necessary, too.

Corn, for example, is low on the amino acid *tryptophane* and lacking the amino acid *lysine*. When processed corn forms the main item in a diet, as it did in many parts of the South, a severe dietary deficiency can occur. Pellagra developed in parts of the Southern states soon after processed corn began to be used. It was discovered that there was nothing wrong with the corn, but that it was deficient as a food and that this deficiency could cause disease. Pellagra is the result of a niacin deficiency and the amino acid tryptophane changes into niacin—which is one of the B vitamins—in the body.

It is interesting to note that the American Indians and some of the early settlers upon occasion lived quite healthfully on a diet of corn and beans as their protein source. An understanding of amino acids, however, makes it clear why. Beans supply the acids lacking in corn; they themselves lack the amino acid *methionine.* The two foods form complete proteins.

How many grams of protein should you eat daily for optimum health? Let's say you have an egg for breakfast, a slice of cheese in a sandwich for lunch, and a serving of roast beef for dinner. That's 6 plus 6, plus perhaps 18. That's 30 grams. Is that enough? The Food and Nutrition Board of the National Research Council doesn't think so.

If you're under three years old, you should have 40 grams a day. If you're between four and six, you should be having 50 grams per day. If you're age seven to nine, add 10 more grams. And if you're ten to twelve, 70 grams daily is recommended. For girls thirteen to fifteen (the years of greatest need), it increases to 80 grams. From sixteen to twenty, 75 grams are recommended. If you're a woman over twenty, you should be eating at least 60 grams of protein daily, or twice as much as the above menu. Boys in the thirteen to fifteen age group should have 85 grams daily; from sixteen to twenty, 100 grams daily are recommended. Men over twenty should eat at least 70 grams daily.

Cheese and eggs and meat and milk are expensive. Health food stores carry excellent sources of complete proteins which cost much less. Try buying brewer's yeast and mixing it into fruit or vegetable juices.

Buy powdered skim milk. Two-thirds cup of the instant contains 18 grams of complete proteins. Two-thirds cup of the noninstant contains 35 grams.

Use wheat germ. In addition to its other nutritional values, it's an excellent source of proteins. One-half cup contains 24 complete proteins.

Or buy soy flour and bake with it. One cup contains 60 grams of complete proteins.

Carbohydrates

Carbohydrates are a second classification of foods. We usually think of them as fattening, and because of the national problem of dieting, which has been caused largely by poor nutrition, we've come to think of all carbohydrates as equally full of calories and, if weight is a problem, to be avoided.

There are two kinds of carbohydrates. Sugars and starch. All starch is changed into sugar in the body. There are some foods, however, which, although high in starch content, contain valuable nutrients. The potato is one. The banana is another.

Carbohydrates are fuel foods and a source of energy. Plants, through the process of photosynthesis, transform carbon, hydrogen, and oxygen into simple sugars. Then, within the plant, these sugars are grouped together into starches. These starches are stored in the stems, flowers, roots, and seeds of plants.

The starches can't be used by the body. They must be broken down into a sugar called *glucose.* When too much sugar is eaten, the blood sugar level rises quickly but then drops quickly, leaving you with a feeling of fatigue.

A meal where protein and some fat is eaten, along with some carbohydrate or sugar, raises the blood sugar level more slowly and the level of energy is maintained for a longer time. It takes fats and proteins longer to be digested; the sugar is absorbed more slowly by the body.

The body needs some sugar; what it doesn't need is an entire diet of sugar. We eat far more sugar than we realize. It's possible to eat one or even two cups of sugar a day and not realize that you've eaten it. Almost every food we eat supplies natural sugar or potential sugar in one form or another. The body uses what it needs for energy; the rest gets stored as fat.

Fruits are our best source of natural sugar. They're classified according to the percentage of sugar they contain. Some fruit should be eaten daily—for its vitamin and mineral content and for the water and roughage it supplies.

If you're counting calories, it's helpful to know which fruits are low in sugar content. You can vary your diet within that group and get a balance of vitamins and minerals. Most fruits contain vitamins A and C, but the amounts differ. The citrus fruits are probably the richest source of vitamin C.

Fruits with 7 percent sugar include the strawberry, watermelon, lemon, and grapefruit. Those in the 10 percent to 15 percent group include the cantaloupe, orange, peach, pineapple, apple, cherry, grape, and pear.

Bananas, fresh figs, and plums are higher in sugar, containing as much as 20 percent. Dried fruits are as high as 75 percent sugar.

Most fruits contain simple sugars, which dissolve easily.

Fats

Some fat is also necessary in the diet. A certain amount of fat produces more energy than an equal amount of sugar. Fats combine with phosphorus to form every cell. Fats are made up of the same substances as starches, carbon, hydrogen, and oxygen. They're usually found combined with protein or carbohydrates. They're either solid or liquid, depending on the fatty acids they contain.

There's been much publicity about saturated and unsaturated fats lately. Unsaturated fats are sometimes called vitamin F. There are three of them, although one—linoleic acid— has been getting most of the publicity. It's the one we need the most.

Fats are broken down by digestion into fatty acids. The body, interestingly enough, can make most of these acids from sugar. But there are three it can't make: linoleic, which is considered an essential nutrient, and arachidonic and linolenic acids which are both important to good health.

The principal sources of these fatty acids are natural vegetable oils. Corn, soybean, and cottonseed oils are high, containing anywhere from 30 percent to 70 percent linoleic acid. Safflower oil, which has had such a vogue and rightfully so, contains 85 percent to 90 percent. In the animal fats and in hydrogenated cooking fats, there is very little fatty acid.

What are hydrogenated fats? Why should we avoid them? Why is unhydrogenated peanut butter good for you, the commercial hydrogenated type not?

Fatty acids are formed like chains. Some have links that are open to which other substances can be easily added. When oxygen is added, the fat becomes rancid. If hydrogen is added, the fat becomes more solid. The body needs the unfilled links, which it can combine with other nutrients.

For commercial purposes, fats are hydrogenated. In the process, the links are closed by the addition of hydrogen. Oxygen can't cause rancidity, and the hydrogenated fat keeps longer. But it isn't very good for you.

Surprisingly enough, eating too little fat is probably a cause of overweight. If you're deficient in this essential nutrient, you may be drinking too much water. Adding fat to your diet will probably cause you to shed some pounds.

Also, when the fatty acids are lacking, the body apparently changes sugar to fat more rapidly than normal. Not a very cheering thought. The body seems in a hurry to supply the fat that you haven't supplied it with. And, when this happens, your blood sugar level drops quickly, causing you to be hungry.

For optimum health, we should eat at least a tablespoon of unsaturated vegetable oils each day. Sesame oil, soybean oil, and sunflower oil are as high in the essential unsaturated fatty acids as safflower oil. Buy freshly pressed oils, keep them tightly covered, and store them in a cool place.

Vitamins

Vitamins and minerals are the regulators of the body processes. We don't need vitamins for fuel, since that is supplied by the fats and carbohydrates. They are essential for health and growth, however. Vitamins have such specific uses that one of them can't replace or act for another.

Vitamins were first discovered around the turn of the century, although it had long been suspected that there were certain vital substances in foods. The idea that a deficiency might actually cause a disease, however, is recent. Scurvy, rickets, and beriberi had been known for centuries. In 1882, a surgeon-general of the Japanese Navy—Kanehiro Takaki—reduced the number of beriberi cases among naval crews by adding meat and vegetables to their diet of rice.

A Dutch medical officer in the East Indies, Christiaan Eijkman, studied beriberi in prison camps, and about 1900 he and a co-worker showed that people who ate polished rice developed beriberi. What was removed from polished rice? The hulls. Those who ate the rice, hulls and all, did not develop the disease. What, they wondered, was in rice hulls?

Experiments to isolate this antiberiberi factor were conducted, and in 1912 a Polish biochemist working in London succeeded. He thought that the substance, which still wasn't quite pure, belonged to a class of chemical compounds called amines and named it *vitamine*. The word *amine* meaning essential to life.

More work was done that clearly showed that there were substances, called "accessory food factors" which were found in certain foods and were essential for growth and normal development.

The letter "e" was dropped from vitamine, and all substances of this type, as yet undifferentiated, were known as vitamins.

At first it was thought that there were only two vitamins—a fat-soluble vitamin, and a water-soluble vitamin.

Then an American biochemist, Elmer J. McCollum, showed that the fat-soluble vitamin was actually a mixture of vitamins.

We know these now as:

Vitamin A

Vitamin D

Vitamin E

Vitamin K

An American physician, Joseph Goldberger, showed that the water-soluble vitamin was also a mixture.

These have been named:

Vitamin C

The B-complex vitamins

Fat-soluble vitamins dissolve in fat; water-soluble vitamins dissolve in water. That's why vitamin C and the B-complex vitamins are not stored in the body. That's why cooking vegetables removed the vitamin C—they promptly dissolve in the water, which, if we're not aware, are thrown away.

Other vitamins have been identified—vitamin P and vitamin U—and scientists believe that still others may be discovered.

How are we supposed to get these substances that are essential to our health and well-being—that regulate our body processes. Two ways. The first, and the best way, is to eat those foods in which they occur naturally. The second, and sometimes the necessary way, is to take vitamins separately. We can buy preparations of pure vitamins which contain either a single vitamin or a combination of several vitamins.

Vitamin A was the first fat-soluble vitamin to be discovered. What does vitamin A do for us? It aids in the building and growth of body cells. It's found in fish liver oils and is particularly important to growing children. The rest of us need it, too. It helps build resistance to infection, helps keep the skin healthy, and helps vision. If you have trouble seeing in a dim light, you probably aren't getting enough vitamin A.

Vitamin A itself occurs only in animals. However, there are several substances in plants that are converted into vitamin A by the body. These plant substances are called carotenes or provitamins. If you're eating carrots or spinach or sweet potatoes, you're getting some of this vitamin. Milk, liver, and egg yolk contain some, as do green and yellow vegetables. The richest source is fish liver oils.

Vitamin D is known as the "sunshine" vitamin. It's a group of about ten fat-soluble vitamins that prevent rickets. Scientists believe that vitamin D_3 forms in the skin when the body is exposed to sunlight.

Vitamin D is not found plentifully in foods. Fish liver oils are the best source. It should be present for calcium and phosphorus to be used properly.

Other sources of vitamin D are irradiated milk and all irradiated animal foodstuffs.

Vitamin E is the fertility vitamin. This is also a fat-soluble vitamin. It was discovered in 1922 in wheat germ oil.

It has been found in other foods, but not in great quantity. In 1939 the pure vitamin E was isolated and the synthetic vitamin E (tocopherol) was made. But the same effects were not achieved with the synthetic as with the wheat germ. So it is generally thought that, like honey and other natural foods, there is some substance in wheat germ that remains nature's secret.

The discovery of vitamin E was more evidence connecting white refined flour with the degenerative diseases which people seem to have been developing within the last fifty years.

It is estimated that our intake of vitamin E before grain was milled was 150 grams. Now it is thought to be around 7 grams.

Vitamin E is found in the oils of all grains, nuts, and seeds. However, it is lost during exposure to air or heat, freezing and storage.

To be sure of getting a good supply of this important vitamin, buy nuts, or fresh wheat germ, cold-pressed oils, or stone-ground, whole-wheat breads and cereals.

Vitamin E is thought to be essential for reproduction and for virility.

Vitamin K is another fat-soluble vitamin. It's essential for the clotting of blood and has cured high blood pressure in animals. The intestinal bacteria in the body produce it. The diet should be adequate in milk and unsaturated fatty acids. Vitamin K is rather abundant in food. It's found in green leafy vegetables, spinach, alfalfa, cabbage, kale, and cauliflower.

Vitamin P is also known as bioflavonoids. It occurs in food with vitamin C. It helps strengthen the capillaries, and the best source of it is the peel and pulp of citrus fruits. Unless you're eating the peel of an organically grown orange, however, you may be getting a dose of insecticides, some artificial coloring, and perhaps some wax.

Vitamin U If you like cabbage juice, you're in luck. That's why it's named "U." People with ulcers were given cabbage juice to drink and all improved quickly. This vitamin is very sensitive to heat and is therefore not found in cooked foods to any extent. Cabbage juice is the best source. It's also found in unpasteurized milk, celery, fresh greens, and cereal grasses.

Vitamin C is a well-known vitamin. What is not so well known is that we may get much less than we think we do. Vitamin C is a water-soluble vitamin, which means that it's difficult for the body to store and must be supplied every day in the diet.

If you bruise easily, it's a sign your vitamin C intake may be low. Vitamin C holds all the cells of the body together. It's necessary for healthy blood vessels and sound bones and teeth. If you're eating the Puerto Rican cherry, you are getting the highest concentration of vitamin C known. If not, citrus fruits are a good source of vitamin C—as are tomatoes, raw cabbage, strawberries, and cantaloupe.

Rose hips are an excellent source of this vitamin. Try rose hip tea. It has a delicious, slightly lemony flavor. Sprouted grains are also very high in vitamin C.

Scurvy has been a problem to man since pre-Christian times. The Romans wrote of it, and there were many cases during the Crusades. But sea-going men seemed to be particularly susceptible. To combat the problem during World War I, England planted fresh gardens all over the world wherever troops were stationed. During the Second World War, to combat the shortage of citrus fruits, the British sprouted grains and made rose hip extract.

Sprouts and products made from rose hips are available in health food stores. When rich, natural sources are available, why not take advantage of them?

The Vitamin B Complex

This is a group of more than fifteen water-soluble vitamins.

Vitamin B_1 is also known as thiamine. It prevents and cures beriberi, a disease of the nervous system, but all of the B vitamins are considered essential for healthy nerves. Vitamin B_1 contains sulphur and nitrogen. Brewer's yeast is particularly rich in B vitaminss and is a good source of B_1. Meats contain it, especially pork. It's also found in soybeans, nuts, peas, and green vegetables.

Alike vitamin A, B_1 is needed for growth. B_1 is part of the process involved in changing carbohydrates into energy. If your appetite is poor, B_1 will help as it will help with fatigue.

Riboflavin was originally called vitamin G and then B_2. It's necessary for healthy skin and growth, for proper functioning of the eyes. B_2 also promotes the body's use of oxygen.

Yeast contains B_2. It's also found in milk, in liver—which is rich in all the B vitamins, including B_{12} —in eggs, poultry, and in fish, and some is found in green and leafy vegetables.

Niacin is also called nicotinic acid. Niacin helps prevent pellagra. It's also essential for growth and for the proper use of oxygen in the body.

It's particularly necessary, because without it, thiamine and riboflavin can't function properly in the body.

Lean meats, whole-grain cereals and breads, and green vegetables are good sources of niacin. Milk and eggs don't contain much niacin but they do contain the amino acid tryptophane—which is converted into niacin by the body.

Vitamin B_{12} contains cobalt. It's not known what all of the things are that B_{12} does. But it is known that injections of tiny amounts of this vitamin help in treating pernicious anemia. Liver is an excellent source of B_{12}. While the "wonder foods" such as brewer's yeast, yogurt, and wheat germ are rich sources of the B vitamins generally, liver is the best source of B_{12}. There is also B^{12} in eggs, milk, meat, and other animal proteins.

Other B complex vitamins include B_6 known as pyridoxine; pantothenic acid; biotin; folic acid; para-aminobenzoic acid; inositol; and choline. Folic acid was first named for foliage because it was first isolated from spinach leaves and is also found in uncooked green vegetables.

Some nutritionists feel that with the widespread use of processed foods, the fifteen or more B vitamins are so little supplied in most diets that almost everyone is deficient in them. Only a few generations ago, even the poorest people were rich in these vitamins. Today, even the wealthiest probably don't get enough.

It's ironic to think that at the time the B vitamins were being discovered, man was busy removing them from his food. The improper milling of grain removes the germ—and with it the B vitamins. It used to be that every food made from whole grain—breads, cereals—was rich in these vitamins. Molasses used to be *the* sweetener. It, too, is rich in the B complex. To make it more of a problem, eating refined sugar increases the need for B vitamins in the system.

It is possible that there is no food eaten daily which supplies a sufficient amount of these vitamins. If you're not willing to risk it, liver, brewer's yeast, wheat germ, rice polish, and yogurt are good sources. The B vitamins are needed equally by all parts of the body. All of them are needed together; eating them separately causes a deficiency in the others.

The "enrichment" of white bread by adding one or two of the B vitamins may not only be inadequate, continued eating of "enriched" white bread could cause deficiencies. The lack of B vitamins may affect your nerves, heart, digestion, tissues, and general morale. If you're supplementing your protein intake with wheat germ, brewer's yeast, or yogurt, you're adding B vitamins to your diet, too.

Minerals

If minerals are not in the soil, they cannot possibly be in the plant. There are other factors involved in growing healthy foods—but the nutritive value is affected directly by the condition of the soil. In some parts of the United States, iodine, for example, is completely lacking and must be supplied in the diet. Iodized salt was developed to meet that need.

Calcium is perhaps the best known of the minerals. It is sometimes referred to as the "lullaby" mineral. What is not so well-known is the part that phosphorus plays in the absorption of calcium by the body. We need large amounts of calcium—eating calcium-rich foods, along with the other essential nutrients, gives us calm nerves and a serene disposition.

Raw milk is an excellent source of calcium. In milk, calcium is combined with phosphorus. Green leafy vegetables are also an excellent source of this important mineral.

Phosphorus, the pure chemical phosphorus, is poisonous, yet food phosphorus used in the body is not toxic and combines with calcium. It acts as a hardening agent for bones and teeth and is necessary to the life processes of every cell. Phosphorus, calcium, and vitamin D are interdependent.

Also, be careful that you don't increase by large quantities your intake of such B-vitamin—rich foods as liver, yeast, and wheat germ without supplementing your diet with a calcium salt—either calcium lactate or calcium gluconate. The liver, yeast, and wheat germ are high in phosphorus but deficient in calcium. If, however, you're eating a well-balanced diet including milk and yogurt, there probably will be no difficulty. If you feel unusually nervous, you'll know that the excess phosphorus has taken calcium from your system since it has not been supplied in your diet.

Moderation would seem to be the key.

Iron   Every cell depends on iron for its oxygen. Anemia is associated with an iron deficiency. Iron has been lost in the refining of breads, cereals, and sugar. Blackstrap molasses is extremely rich in iron. Brewer's yeast and wheat germ are good sources. Green, leafy vegetables contain iron, as do fresh fruits, most notably the apricot.

Iodine   The need for small amounts of iodine in the body is quite well known. The thyroid gland was discovered in 1895, and since then, there has been an awareness of the importance iodine plays in the proper functioning of this gland.

Ocean fish and other seafoods are good sources of iodine.

Seaweed is an excellent source, and has been and is being used in other countries for food. We're beginning to discover it as a food source, and it can be purchased in a health food store—it's usually known as kelp.

Iodized salt contains the amount of iodine that occurs naturally in unrefined ocean salt.

Potassium, sodium, and chlorine are three nutrients important to the body, and large amounts of them are needed daily. The sodium and the chlorine are obtained in ordinary table salt. Potassium is found in potatoes and leafy vegetables, fruits, as well as whole grains, nuts, and meats.

Chlorine is also found in raw meat, milk, leafy greens, sea greens, tomatoes, and radishes in good amounts. Sodium is found in muscle meats and in all vegetables. In other words, if you're eating plenty of leafy greens, whole grains and meats, you should be getting an ample supply.

It's not enough for these three just to be adequate, however. The sodium and potassium must be in balance. As people eat fewer and fewer vegetables and fruits, their possible sources of potassium are less.

Unfortunately we are eating more and more salt—sometimes from sources we aren't aware of. Sodium nitrates are used as food preservatives, and we get additional sodium from any number of the hundreds of food additives in which it is used. Sodium is a balancing mineral as is potassium. Sodium neutralizes citric acid, for example. Working together, the sodium and potassium extract nourishment from the blood stream for the cells.

The digestive juices in the body use chlorine—hydrochloric acid is one of these juices.

Trace Minerals

The trace minerals, which we've been hearing a lot about, are minerals that exist in small amounts but that are necessary for good health. What are they?

Cobalt is a part of Vitamin B_{12}. Liver is an excellent source.

Copper is essential before iron can be utilized. Copper is found in some of the enzyme formations in the body. If only unrefined foods are eaten, the intake of copper will probably be adequate. It's found in liver and green leafy vegetables if they were grown on fertile soils, and in whole grains, and dried fruits.

Zinc Nuts and green, leafy vegetables, if grown on healthy soils, are good sources of zinc. If you're eating shellfish, you can probably be sure you're getting a supply. Zinc has a number of important functions in the body; it's present in all the tissues, and the male hormone is not produced without zinc. Zinc is essential for the action of many enzymes and for the body's use of proteins.

Manganese is another mineral needed for the activity of various enzymes. It's found in wheat germ, nuts, green, leafy vegetables, and whole-grain cereals.

Chromium is needed before the body can use sugar. Chromium is often lacking in soils that are either worn out or have been fertilized with chemicals lacking this mineral.

The above materials, then, are the essential nutrients: the amino acids of the proteins, natural sugars from either fresh fruits or starches as they occur in natural foods, the essential, unsaturated fatty acids, and the important vitamins and minerals.

Planned Nutrition

Is there a convenient way to know if we're eating a nourishing daily diet? Choose your foods from among these groups, being sure to include some of each.

Proteins
Milk, powdered milk, buttermilk, yogurt, cheese
Meats, poultry, fish, eggs
Soybeans, soybean flour

Carbohydrates
Fresh fruits and vegetables—corn, peas, lima beans, potatoes
Whole-grain breads and cereals

Fats
Natural vegetable oils—soybean, safflower, corn, sesame
Nuts and unhydrogenated nut butters

Vitamins

VITAMIN A
Fish liver oils
Milk, liver, egg yolk
Green and yellow vegetables

VITAMIN D
Fish liver oil
Irradiated milk
Sunshine

VITAMIN E
Wheat germ oil
Fresh wheat germ or stone-ground wheat breads and
cereals
Cold-pressed oils
Nuts

VITAMIN P
Peel and pulp of citrus fruits

VITAMIN U
Raw cabbage juice
Unpasteurized milk
Celery, fresh greens, cereal grasses

VITAMIN C
Citrus fruits
Tomatoes, raw cabbage, strawberries, cantaloupe
Puerto Rican cherry
Rose hips

B VITAMINS
In general: brewer's yeast, wheat germ, rice polish, yogurt

B_1
Brewer's yeast, meats
Soybeans, nuts, peas
Green vegetables

Riboflavin (B_2)
Milk, liver, eggs, poultry, fish
Green and leafy vegetables

Niacin
Lean meats
Whole-grain cereals and breads
Green vegetables

Vitamin B_{12}
Liver
Eggs, milk, meat, and other animal proteins

Minerals

CALCIUM
Raw milk, yogurt
Green leafy vegetables

PHOSPHORUS
Liver, yeast, wheat germ
Milk, eggs, cheese, meats

IRON
Blackstrap molasses
Green, leafy vegetables
Fresh fruits

IODINE
Seafoods
Kelp
Iodized salt

POTASSIUM, SODIUM, AND CHLORINE

Potassium
Potatoes, green, leafy vegetables, fruits
Nuts, meats, whole grains

Sodium
Table salt, muscle meats
All vegetables

Chlorine
Table salt, raw meat, milk
Leafy greens, sea greens, tomatoes

TRACE MINERALS

Cobalt
Liver

Copper
Liver, whole grains
Dried fruits, green, leafy vegetables

Zinc
Nuts, green, leafy vegetables

Manganese
Wheat germ, nuts, green, leafy vegetables
Whole-grain cereals

Chromium
Unrefined foods grown on healthy soils

To Cook or Not To Cook?

Not to cook whenever possible. Cooking destroys enzymes. Cooking destroys many vitamins. Raw foods are more effective as bulk than are cooked foods.

Slow heat and a little water or none at all is the best way to cook. Cooking does make the starch in vegetables more digestible. Waterless cooking is the best—using durable, sheet aluminum utensils. The biggest loss of vitamins and minerals occurs with the old-fashioned method of cooking—water covering the vegetable and the lid left slightly off to allow passage of steam. If we're not careful, the water we simmer our vegetables in will be more healthful than the vegetables.

If you don't have the utensils for waterless cooking, use about one-half cup of water, bring it to a quick boil at high heat and then keep it at a slow boil until the vegetables are done.

HANDBOOK OF HEALTH FOODS

CHEESE

Cheese is one of man's earliest foods and among the most nourishing. It's not known when the first primitive cheese was made—probably some four thousand years ago.

It was almost certainly accidental. Some say it happened when an Arab was traveling across the desert with milk carried in a pouch he had made of a sheep's stomach. By nightfall, the milk had separated into a liquid and a solid. Rennet had caused the separation. This is a substance found in a sheep's stomach which causes milk to curdle.

Cheeses may be divided into two categories, according to how the curd is formed. Rennet is used in the first group, and most cheeses are formed by this method. In the second category, curds are formed by lactic acid. Cream cheese is one of the most important in this group.

Cheese is an excellent source of protein. The protein part of milk is the casein. When rennet comes in contact with milk, the casein coagulates into a semisolid mass. This is called curd. The water liquid that is left is whey, which is what Little Miss Muffett sat on her tuffet eating.

Cheese is also classified as hard or soft. The difference between hard and soft cheese depends on several things. One is the amount of moisture, or whey, left in the curd. Another is the bacteria or mold used to produce a characteristic flavor. And yet a third is the method used in curing.

Cheddar and Swiss are common types of hard cheese. Cream, Brie, Camembert are classified as soft cheeses. Brick, Muenster and bleu cheese are among those that may be described as semisoft.

Some cheeses may have aphrodisiac qualities. "Have Roquefort with a fine Chambertin wine, and you'll be ready for love," wrote Casanova.

There seems to be a possible connection between fungi and virility. Mushrooms are fungi and truffles are fungi. The legendary aphrodisiac qualities of truffles are well-documented. Fungi like cheese. Thus the connection of fungi and virility to mold-ripened cheese.

It was probably several thousand years after primitive forms of cheese were discovered that flavor was added by molds. And again, probably by chance.

Legend has it that it happened in France, near the little town of Roquefort. It's a simple legend. A young sheep herder, taking shelter in a cave from a sudden downpour, left his lunch of bread and cheese. Several weeks later he returned to find the bread crumbled but the cheese still there, with veins of a blue green mold in it. History might have been different had our shepherd not been hungry, and adventurous, too. And they began bringing their cheese to the caves around Roquefort.

The mold that causes the blue green veins is present everywhere. We call it now penicillium Roquefort. So it was inevitable that as the fame of the Roquefort cheese spread, people elsewhere would develop similar cheeses. However, there is a unique factor about the caves at Roquefort. A series of cracks and crevices lead both up to the top of the mountain and down to an underground river. As a result, there is a steady flow of cool, moist air through the caves. This keeps the temperature at a constant 50°F and the humidity at 95 percent.

It wasn't until 1918 that we were able by trial and error to guess what those conditions were and duplicate them. So it remained a secret for two thousand years.

Imitations were inevitable in those early days, and the cheese-makers of Roquefort applied to the King of France for help. Charles VI ruled that only cheeses made near the town of Roquefort could be called by that name.

Later, laws were passed to continue the protection, and today a French regulation still limits the use of the name. Bleu cheese is the name given to other similar varieties of these blue green, mold-ripened cheeses.

All bleu cheeses are made with the same mold. However, not all are made with the same kind of milk. In the United States, either cow's or goat's milk is used. In France, the true Roquefort, of course, is made from sheep's milk.

If you're in France, visit the town of Roquefort when the cheese-making is in process. It is still made in some twenty-five caves in the mountainside and is a colorful local industry. Three hundred dairies produce the curd used in the cheese, and the entire town of 1,300 is engaged in the business of cheese-making.

There are cheeses made in other countries which have the same blue green mold as the French Roquefort and bleu.

Gorgonzola was originated in Italy in 879A.D. It helped make Italy the cheese-making center of Europe for the next two hundred years.

Stilton, a cheese made by the English, has never been successfully duplicated by any other people. It's a cream-colored cheese, with the same blue green penicillium roquefortus veins that give flavor to Roquefort and Gorgonzola. Stilton's taste is milder than either, however.

Blue-veined cheeses in other countries include: Greek *Kpoanisti*, Norwegian *Gammelost*, and Swiss *Paglia*.

Camembert is a different type of mold-ripened cheese. The molds grow above ground. Camembert, like Roquefort, was created in the village for which it is named. According to legend, Napoleon visited the town and, liking the cheese, asked its name. He was told that it had none, so he named it Camembert.

Brie is a similar cheese, made in another region of France.

Limburger owes its odor to surface yeast and bacteria. It originated in Belgium. *Poona* is a similar cheese developed in New York State. It is a milder cheese.

Bel paese, meaning beautiful country and referring to Italy, is also milder. The surface molds are allowed to remain only a short time.

Port du Salut is another French cheese—made by Trappist monks at the abbey at Port du Salut. They have kept their methods secret for nearly a hundred years.

Neufchatel is sometimes described as a cream cheese with character. *American Neufchatel* differs in flavor, again because Americans tend to prefer milder cheeses and the molds are not allowed to remain as long.

Another soft cheese is cooked cheese, sometimes called "cup" cheese or "Pennsylvania pot cheese." It is still prepared in homes as well as in dairies; one of the few cheeses that are. It's made of milk from which the cream has been removed, and so is lower in calories. A heavy mold provides a delicious flavor. In texture, it resembles Camembert.

Thus mold-ripening cheese enhances flavor, and, who knows, may increase virility. Aside from these benefits, cheese is extremely nutritious. Cheese is a superior source of protein. Cheese contains more amino acids, in more abundance, than do vegetable proteins. Cheese contains complete proteins. All cheese is rich in calcium and phosphorus.

Processed cheeses should be avoided. They contain hydrogenated fats. Old-fashioned cheeses do not. As an "ancient and honorable" product, it comes in a variety of kinds and flavors. Experiment. Find the cheese that best suits your taste — hard or soft, mild or tart, made from cow, goat, or sheep's milk.

NUTS

The chief value of nuts lies in their protein content. Nuts are also a good source of fat, and, although they are not particularly rich in vitamins, they contain carbohydrates and are rich in minerals. Their mineral composition resembles that of cereals, peas, and beans.

It has been said that nuts are the quintessence of nutriment—"the chef-d'oeuvre of Nature"—that they supply for a given weight nearly twice the amount of nutrients supplied by any other food product.

Nuts are sometimes considered a seed food, although they are actually a one-seeded fruit consisting of a kernel in a woody shell. As a fruit, nuts are considered dry-stone fruits—differing from such stone fruits as the cherry or peach.

Nuts were probably among the first foods eaten by early man. The almond is mentioned in the Bible, and both almonds and walnuts have been eaten since ancient times.

The Romans, noted for their love of good food, valued the almond, and, interestingly enough, called almonds "Greek nuts." Which suggests, of course, that they came from Greece. They have been cultivated all along the Mediterranean coast. Almonds and walnuts were also eaten by the ancient Chinese.

It is thought that walnuts were first cultivated in Persia, since the Greeks called it *persicon* (Persian tree). The Greeks and Romans planted walnuts on the shores of the Mediterranean. Spanish padres first brought walnuts to California, but it wasn't until 1867 that they were planted commercially.

Almonds are an edible, nut-like seed of a fruit like a peach. A milk is made from them which has a high protein content. Almond meal or paste is used in cakes and candies.

Walnuts are a roundish, edible nut, with a two-lobed seed. They have an acid reaction in the body and should be used with milk or other alkaline food.

Both almonds and walnuts contain excellent, though not complete proteins.

Millions in the tropics depend on nuts as their staple food, a fact which is perhaps not generally realized. There are probably hundreds of lesser-known tropical nuts eaten in the locality where they grow. Some tropical nuts have gained popularity in other countries, mainly during the last several hundred years. These include cashews, pistachios, Brazil nuts, and coconuts. The pecan is our best native nut; American Indians used nuts from pines, horse chestnuts, and oaks.

The cashew tree is a tropical tree in Brazil. The cashew fruit is shaped like a pear and the nut is attached to the end of it. The nut looks like a large kidney bean, and inside is what we call the "cashew" nut.

The *cashew* was taken from Brazil by Portuguese explorers in the sixteenth century, first to Goa and then all over the tropics. We eat cashews either plain or salted, or put into candies or other confections. In the tropics, however, they may be curried or stewed or mixed with bean flour and fried in oil.

The *pistachio* nut grows on a small tree of the cashew family. It originally grew in Turkestan and Afghanistan. Now it's cultivated on the Mediterranean coast, in Asia Minor, and Persia. In India, they use it in a variety of sweetmeats. In Turkey it's one of the ingredients of Turkish "rahat loukoum." In this country we can buy the little green-flecked nut packaged—they are rather expensive—or we may eat it in ice cream and other confections.

The *coconut* is said to be the most widely used tropical nut in this country. It is also the fruit of a tropical tree—the coconut palm. Because they grow so close to the sea, they're rich in minerals. They have a natural bulk, unsaturated fatty acids, and they're high in vitamins. You can buy them shredded or fresh when in season.

The *Brazil nut* is an interesting nut. Originally from Brazil, as its name implies, it was first exported to Europe in the seventeenth century. It did not, for some reason, become popular in Brazil until rather recently. But it ranked third after coffee and rubber as an export in the nineteenth century.

One of the most interesting things about Brazil nuts is the trees themselves. They stand one hundred and fifty feet high and there are millions of them in the forests of Brazil. They've never been cultivated and they're propagated by the Amazonian hare. The hare gathers up the nuts and buries them. Then, as hares will do, he digs them up and eats them. The few that he forgets about grow into trees.

The nut, or fruit, is about the size of a coconut and weighs from two to four pounds. No one has to pick the fruits. Once a year, high winds snap the fruits from the tall trees and hurl them to the ground. What we know as "Brazil nuts" are the hard, triangular seeds that are packed inside these fruits—anywhere from twelve to twenty-five of them. Brazil nuts are used mainly in confections.

Nuts are a rich source of proteins and carry all of the amino acids. As vegetable proteins, however, they are not considered as "biologically effective" as the animal proteins—which contain more concentrated amounts of the well-known eight amino acids. Nuts are a good source of fat.

Nuts are also a source of the B vitamin, niacin; and vitamin B_1, thiamin, is found in nuts because it is necessary before seeds can sprout.

Vitamin E is found in the oils of nuts. They are one of only a few sources.

Nuts are rich in minerals, provided they have been grown

on good soils and without chemical fertilizers. They are one of the best sources of magnesium; potassium occurs in nuts, and they are a rich source of zinc and manganese.

The *peanut*, a highly nutritious food, is not actually a nut. Like soybeans and peas, it is a legume. This vine of the pea family has branches which bury themselves in the ground as the plant matures, forming peanuts within its pods.

Originally the peanut came from Brazil and is thought to have been carried first to West Africa by the Portuguese and then to other parts of the world. Its value as a cheap, nutritious food was recognized in India where, at one time, as many as eight million acres were used for its cultivation. In this country, the work of Dr. George Washington Carver, the noted Negro scientist, resulted in the production of over three thousand by-products from the peanut, and his Institute at Tuskegee became world-renowned.

Peanuts, also called monkey nuts or ground nuts, are an excellent source of protein. They are rich in minerals and contain large amounts of the B vitamins and vitamin E. They're a good source of oil which contains the essential unsaturated fatty acids.

Peanuts are most healthful when eaten raw or lightly roasted.

RAW CERTIFIED MILK

Milk is an excellent source of complete proteins. What are the advantages of raw certified milk as compared to pasteurized milk? We tend to think of unpasteurized milk as unsafe; the process of pasteurization was developed in order to destroy harmful bacteria in milk by heating.

Unfortunately, the process also destroys our best health builders. Raw "certified" milk is considered safe to drink. Cows have to be fed a very rich green-feed diet (fifty pounds a day) to make milk of such high quality that it can pass the low bacteria count and be classified as certified. The health of the cows has to be excellent to have this high quality milk.

Certified milk was conceived more than sixty years ago by a practicing physician, Dr. Henry L. Coit, of Newark, New Jersey. In 1893, Dr. Coit laid down seventy rules for the production of certified milk. He organized the first Medical Milk Commission; modern methods and skills have modified his original standards, but his basic plan is still in operation.

Certified milk is clean, fresh, and very nutritious. Nutrition-control for cows producing certified milk begins with the soil and carries through to the actual feeding of the cow. The more nutritious a cow's diet, the more nutritive values there are in her milk. Strict, laboratory control standards of cows' rations assure maximum nutritional values and quality, and special precautions protect the nutritional content and flavor of certified milk.

In a partial reprint from the "National Health Federation Bulletin," certified raw milk is compared point by point with pasteurized milk. Five areas are considered:

Cleanliness
Herd tests in Los Angeles County
Employee health examinations
Nutritional values
Spoilage

Cleanliness   According to this bulletin, milk, to qualify as certified raw milk, is tested daily in the laboratory of the County Milk Commission for bacteria count, whereas, under California State and County law, pasteurized milk is generally tested twice a month.

Herd Test   The regulations differ. Raw milk is tested for a standard plate count of five thousand bacteria per mililiter maximum in order to qualify for certified milk or cream. Pasteurized milk is acceptable with a standard plate count of seventy-five thousand per mililiter bacteria count before pasteurization and fifteen thousand per mililiter maximum after pasteurization, with twenty-five thousand per mililiter for cream.

For certified raw milk, the coliform bacteria count may not exceed ten per mililiter. The requirement for pasteurized milk after pasteurization is the same.

Certified raw milk is tested once a week for anaerobic. *No test* is required for pasteurized milk. The bulletin states that there have been no pathogens (bacteria that cause disease) in fifty-six years of record. Pasteurized milk is usually safe from pathogens.

A streptococci test once a month is required for certified raw milk—no test for streptococci is required for pasteurized milk.

Milk contains what might be called nature's antiseptic—friendly acid-forming bacteria. These retard the growth of invading organisms (bacteria). So the bacterial growth in certified raw milk increases very slowly.

The minimum pasteurization temperature is usually 165° to 167° for twenty-two seconds or longer. Usually the higher the bacteria count, the higher the pasteurization temperature. But pasteurizing does not remove dirt, dead bacteria, or bacterially produced toxins from milk.

Certified raw milk usually keeps for two weeks when under constant refrigeration and it will sour. Commercial milk, as most of us have observed, gradually turns rancid in a few days and then decomposes. The bacteria growth is rapid.

Certified milk is not available in all parts of the country. In Los Angeles County, a veterinarian, designated by the County Milk Commission, examines the cows every sixty days. A ring test is made on the milk for brucella once a month. According to regulations, if a cow had brucellosis, it would be removed from the herd *at once*. It takes three months from the time of a cow's infection to the time that brucella appears in the milk.

Under state and county law, however, which regulates the inspection of cows whose milk is pasteurized, all dairy herds in the Los Angeles, Orange, and Ventura Counties receive only three ring tests for brucellosis annually. In case test results are suspicious, a complete herd blood test is made and any reactors are removed.

For those cows whose milk is to be "certified," a tuberculosis skin test is made every six months by a veterinarian; with cows in commercial dairies, the tests are run annually. Again, if reactors are found, additional tests may be required. The sick cows are then, of course, removed.

A herd sanitarian from the County Milk Commission visits a dairy which is producing certified raw milk once a month. There is no visit to other dairy herds.

Employee Health Examinations At a Certified Farm, each

employee is examined once a month. All new employees have complete physical examinations and tests when starting to work on a certified farm. For other farms, the California State and County law requires an examination at the time of employment.

Those working on certified farms have once-a-month throat cultures and examination for streptococcus, and during the year, other tests are made at regular intervals. Another important step to insure disease-free milk. Because of the theory that pasteurization kills germs, *no* examinations of those employees are required except for the initial examination at the time of employment.

Nutritional Values There are many nutritional values in milk, many of which are altered or destroyed by heating—*enzymes, protein, fats, vitamins, carbohydrates,* and *minerals.* Milk contains them all, in varying degrees depending on the source of feed of the cows and the soil in which the feed is grown. In milk from healthy cows, all enzymes are available—catalase, peroxidase, phosphatase—in addition to the Wulzen (antistiffness) factor and the X factor in tissue repair. Milk that has gone through the heating process called pasteurization has fewer than 10 percent of its enzymes remaining. There is an almost total destruction of enzymes. The Wulzen (antistiffness) nutrition factor is lost and the X factor is also destroyed.

In certified raw milk, protein is 100 percent available, with at least eighteen amino acids, including the eight essential ones.

In pasteurized milk, protein-lysine and tyrosine are altered by heat with serious loss of metabolic availability. This results in making the whole protein complex less available for tissue repair and rebuilding. Anyone for a protein-lysine or tyrosine tablet?

All eighteen fatty acids that occur naturally in healthy

whole milk are metabolically available in certified raw milk, both saturated and unsaturated. An interesting fact: research studies indicate that fats are necessary to metabolize protein and calcium. *All natural protein-bearing foods contain fat.* Fats are altered by heat—especially the essential unsaturated fats.

And what about vitamins? In raw, certified milk, *all vitamins are 100 percent available.*

Vitamin A	Vitamin E
Vitamin D	The B vitamin complex
Vitamin E—metabolically available	Vitamin C—ascorbic acid

Some of the fat-soluble vitamins are classed as unstable, and therefore a loss is caused by heating above blood temperature. This loss can run as high as two-thirds.

Several water-soluble vitamins are affected by heat. Losses on many can run from 38 percent to 80 percent. The loss of vitamin C in the heating process usually exceeds 50 percent.

In raw certified milk, the carbohydrates are easily utilized in metabolism. They are still associated naturally with elements. However, feeding tests have indicated that heat makes some changes in carbohydrates, making them less available metabolically.

The major mineral components in milk are:

calcium	potassium
chlorine	sodium
magnesium	sulphur
phosphorus	

These minerals are all 100 percent metabolically available in healthy milk that has not been heated to high temperatures, and the vital trace minerals, all twenty-four or more, are 100 percent available.

Calcium, one of the major minerals in milk, is altered by heat and the loss may run 50 percent or more depending on the pasteurization temperature.

Losses in the metabolic availability in one mineral means losses in other essential minerals, since one mineral usually acts as a synergist for another element. Sometimes a minute amount of a mineral element restores proper cellular metabolism in repairing defective tissue.

Enzymes serve as leaders in the assimilation of minerals. Since 90 percent of the enzymes are destroyed in pasteurized milk, this means that you may get very little of the needed minerals.

The friendly, protective, acid-forming bacteria in milk are destroyed by heating. These bacteria are a plus-factor for health. Nature works to promote health if the natural balance is allowed to remain.

Pasteurization alters the biochemistry of milk and that includes the alteration of protein compounds and minerals, making them less available or not available at all, depending on the temperatures.

Spoilage Pasteurized milk does not keep as well as clean raw milk because of the destruction of the friendly acid-forming bacteria. There are no regulations for dating or limits set on the age of milk, although the carton may read "fresh."

VEGETABLES

In its wider definition, a vegetable is any plant, as distinguished from animal or inorganic matter. In more common usage, *vegetable* refers to edible plants such as the potato, lettuce, or tomato which are eaten whole or in part in salads or with entrees.

A health food store is not concerned with how big or how small vegetables are. They don't wax them—to look fresher and more nutritious than they are. They don't dye them—to trick you into thinking they are fresher or more colorful than they really are. A health food store sells you vegetables that are highly nutritious, that have been grown on healthy soils, free of pesticides.

There is only one basic food factory—and that's in the green leaves and other green parts of plants. The true fertility of the soil depends largely on trace minerals, of which there are some thirty-two—including iron, cobalt, magnesium, and zinc. That's partly what organic gardening is all about—returning the trace minerals and organic matter that have been removed back to the soil.

When we talk about eating natural foods, we're talking about going back, as best we can, to the vegetables grown in rich, unpoisoned earth, nurtured by rain and sun, with all of nature's nourishment stored in them.

Vegetables are particularly important because of the minerals and vitamins they contain. They are especially rich in such vitamins as A, thiamin, niacin, and C.

Vegetables are also an important source of minerals: calcium, phosphorus, iron.

In addition to potatoes, we should eat daily one green, leafy vegetable and one yellow vegetable. Vegetables give bulk to the diet, which helps the digestive process. They're among the three types of foods we should eat each day: animal foods, providing protein; starchy foods providing carbohydrates; and vegetables—which don't have great caloric or energy-giving value but are excellent for minerals and vitamins and bulk.

Peas and beans are an exception and contain valuable proteins.

The aristocratic asparagus is a native of southern Russia, Poland, and Siberia. It has traveled, through the centuries, from Europe to America where it is grown primarily in California and New Jersey.

The asparagus is a cousin of the orchid. It has a fine, delicate taste. It is used in fashionable dishes such as asparagus vinaigrette, as a table vegetable, sometimes used in soups, and, like the cucumber, in sandwiches—there are 150 varieties of this elegant vegetable.

Asparagus contains a rich abundance of nutritive elements. There is a wealth of vitamins and minerals in this vegetable. When buying asparagus, select straight, firm stalks with the leaves of the spear closely and firmly united and with a maximum of three inches of white base.

Asparagus is particularly rich in vitamin A.

Beets, by contrast, were for a long time considered a lowly food. They were grown in Holland and Germany for centuries. Their use spread to France, and, during a near famine, were often the only food the peasants could get. The French called them *racine de disette*, intending a translation from the German *mangoldwurzel*. However, there was confusion between the German word for beet *(mangold)* and what the French apparently thought they were called *(mangel*—meaning dearth). Dearth translating into the French as *disette*.

When attempts to introduce beets into England were made, the English were put off by the "root of dearth" rather than the correct translation of the German "root of beet," and for years English farmers fed the beet root to stock, refusing to eat it themselves. Gradually, however, the beet became a popular vegetable.

The beet is considered a taproot by botanists—that is, a main root growing downward, from which branch roots spread out. There are various types of beets. The mangold is still generally used as stock food. Sugar beets, of which there are several kinds, are grown primarily in order to refine their sucrose content into white sugar. Garden beets are also high in sucrose, as well as in three other kinds of sugar.

Ideally, beets should be eaten raw. They may be shredded and added to salads or cooked Chinese-fashion in a little oil. If you boil them, keep the skin on, the root on, and as much of the stem as you can. The amount of food value lost in cooking is repeatedly stressed by nutritionists. In boiling beets, this is shown dramatically. There is no question that the beet juice with its minerals and vitamins is being lost in the cooking water—the red color of the water speaks for itself.

Beets are a source of good natural sugar, as well as of minerals and vitamins. Beet greens are particularly rich in vitamin A. However, it should be remembered that they also contain oxalic acid—as does spinach—which connects rapidly with calcium. Oxalates are formed which are then excreted. So don't depend on beet greens exclusively for the greens in your diet.

Brussels sprouts belong to the cabbage family—developed mostly by Dutch gardeners from the wild *brassica maritime.* Sprouts have small cabbagelike heads on their tall stems.

Mustard, radishes, and watercress also belong to—as one nutritionist put it—"this enormous tribe."

The leaves of the cabbage family absorb energy from the

sun. This is done by means of the chlorophyll in their green parts. Chlorophyll comes from the Greek *chloros* meaning green and *phyllon* meaning leaf. It's the green coloring matter in plants which converts carbon dioxide and water into carbohydrates.

Where there is chlorophyll, there is almost always vitamin A. Iron is found, too, in abundance. Vitamin C is present and acts as a catalyst to bring about the changes in the leaf that permit the formation of the carbohydrates or sugar from the carbon dioxide and water. This is what is meant by the "chemical factory" in plant life. The greener the leaf, the more vitamin A, iron, and vitamin C you can expect to find.

Brussels sprouts are a good food for dieters. They're low in calories and they're low in starch.

The cabbage, says the dictionary, is a vegetable with thick leaves, compressed into a round head. The Greeks and Romans ate cabbages at their banquets. The wine flowed freely, and they believed it would keep them from becoming intoxicated. Try it if you like; no studies have been made, but the health-giving qualities of cabbage have been known for a long time.

Foods of the cabbage family have the reputation of being "gassy" and "strong"; anyone who has walked into a kitchen where cabbage was being boiled, can easily understand why. Overdone cabbage is unappetizing; cooking cabbage for a long time or over a slow heat breaks down the sulfur compounds which accounts for the unpleasant odor. To add baking soda to restore the color increases the problem; a bright green color is restored but vitamin C is destroyed.

In the eighteenth century, a famous gourmet remarked: "The English have only three vegetables, and two of them are cabbage." It was being boiled in millions of British homes until it was a soggy mess, and according to an Englishman, "Nowhere is cabbage less tastefully cooked than in Britain."

It wasn't always like that; in twelfth-century England, cabbage was excellent and conformed to the best present-day conservative cooking which retains the valuable mineral salts.

Cabbage is best served crisp and raw. Don't shred it until you're ready to serve it to prevent loss of vitamin C. Use it for slaw or salad. If you do want to cook it, put it still chilled into a little boiling water. Reduce the heat; cover, and cook no longer than eight to ten minutes.

Cabbage is 90 percent water. It contains large amounts of vitamins and minerals, and, with the exception of parsley, is the best source of vitamin C of all vegetables.

Not long ago, scientists at Stanford University found that the juice of cabbage is rich in vitamins K and U. U helps heal stomach ulcers; but you have to drink about a quart of raw cabbage juice a day.

Carrots have been cultivated since very early times. But they weren't held in very high esteem until more recently. Carrots are a plant with a fleshy, edible orange red root. During the latter part of the eighteenth century, they were thought to have healing powers and were made into paste. These powers were probably the result of the vitamins and minerals in carrots—they are particularly rich in the alkaline minerals and especially in carotene.

Carotene is the substance that gives carrots their yellow color. It also becomes vitamin A in the body. Vitamin A is valuable in helping protect against infection. It is also well known as protection against night blindness—the inability to see well in a dim light or after dark.

When vegetables are cut and exposed to air, the losses in vitamin C are high. However, with carrots, a choice needs to be made—probably in favor of their much higher vitamin A content. Studies have shown that when raw or cooked carrots are eaten, only about 2 to 5 percent of the carotene is absorbed by the body, no matter how well they are chewed.

But when carrots are well shredded before eating, from 4 to 36 percent is absorbed. Fresh carrot juice seems to offer optimum benefit from carotene, since in juicing, the cell walls are well broken down.

Winter-grown carrots are lower in carotene; young carrots are more tender but have less sugar and carotene than fully mature ones. Mid-August is the best time for carrots that have been planted in the spring.

Celery derives from the Greek *selinon*, meaning parsley. It's a plant whose crisp stalks are eaten as a vegetable. It's not easy to grow—it needs rich, moist soils and cool temperatures.

Bleaching celery is a common practice and adds nothing to health, since it destroys the chlorophyll and other values. By the blanching process, all of the vitamin A of the celery is destroyed, much of the vitamin C, and a considerable portion of the B vitamins. Pascal celery is green and unbleached.

Organically grown, unbleached celery is very different from the commercial variety—having a delectable and crisp taste. Much of the commercial celery has been stored for a long time and shows it. It's limp and rather tasteless.

Celery is a rich source of vitamins A and B, calcium, sodium, potassium, phosphorus, and iron, and has an alkaline reaction in the body. Celery salt, popular as a seasoning, is dehydrated celery which has been pulverized.

Corn Columbus, searching for a short route to India, and finding America instead, brought back, in place of spices, several new vegetables of which corn is one. Sir Walter Raleigh spoke of this country and its natives who had "corne, which yields them bread; and this with little labor and in abundance. 'Tis called in the Spanish tongue *mahiz.*"

Corn is considered the most valuable, annual food crop in this country. Only a small percentage is used for food and industrial purposes. About 10 percent or less. About half of this is used for cornstarch, corn oil, and feed by-products. Of the rest, about a third is used for corn meal and breakfast cereal, the remainder being used for distilled liquors such as bourbon.

Corn, like wheat, has undergone changes in processing. In early days in this country, corn was "water-ground." The term describes the process by which corn was ground between stones in a mill that was powered by water. The meal that was produced had all the original grain—including the germ. As a result, the meal was highly perishable.

Now corn is milled by the same methods we use to mill flour. All the vital, alive food elements are removed so that the meal will keep indefinitely in storehouses and on grocery shelves.

Corn has been subjected to an "enrichment" program, too, and some of the vitamins and minerals have been put back. These are synthetic and of questionable value. In addition, a substance is added to the vitamins which makes them no longer water soluble, thus protecting them from the various washings the corn goes through, but hopefully leaving them in a state where they can be assimilated by the body.

There is more than nostalgia for old-fashioned water mills. Corn has a high carbohydrate content, about 75 percent. As with wheat, the germ contains most of the vitamins and minerals. The germ is also rich in oil. A fresh ear of sweet corn, newly picked, is nourishing and satisfying.

Corn oil, made from the germ, is a rich source of the unsaturated fatty acid—linoleic acid. And, like other cereals, corn is poor in calcium and rich in phosphorus.

The proteins in corn are about 10 percent of its composition, as compared to wheat which contains a higher percent. One amino acid is lacking entirely—lysine, and there is only a small amount of the amino acid tryptophane. When the whole grain is eaten, the other amino acids tend to make up the deficiency. The disease pellagra, which raged in our Southern states after the new milling processes began to be used, is a dramatic example of what can happen when we tamper with foods. Pellagra is caused by a niacin deficiency, and the processed corn, lacking tryptophane (which changes into niacin in the body) and eaten as the main part of the diet by poorer people where other foods are deficient, caused this disease.

Eggplant is a plant with a large, pear-shaped, purple-skinned fruit, eaten as a vegetable. Its use dates back to early civilizations. It gets its name from certain tropical varieties which are white and small and egg-shaped in appearance. It's a favorite food in Asia, the Mediterranean countries, and Spain. The Near East places it high on its list of delicacies.

As with other "health foods," eggplant is an example of foods that the so-called backward countries have used and enjoyed for centuries, to the benefit of their health.

Eggplant is actually a member of the berry family, and one of the loveliest in coloring. The eggplant seems to be one of the few foods that has escaped the modernization process—its skin is thick enough to repel chemicals, although insecticides and other chemicals are sprayed on it.

Eggplant contains valuable vitamins and minerals and is particularly high in phosphorus.

Lettuce is one of the greens used as the basis for almost every salad. Its use dates back to the Roman Empire, where it was eaten, but with some suspicion. Apparently, lettuce contains laudanum, which is a tincture of opium. The Romans weren't sure how wholesome it was, and thought it made them sleepy. Being great salad eaters, they apparently ate it anyhow, and drank a large, snail shellful of a concoction called oxporon which they made with cummin, ginger, green-rue, nitre, dates, pepper, and honey. This they mixed with vinegar and liquamen.

The Romans, like the French, ate their salads last. So did the English until after the Romans left the British Isles, then, for some reason, it began to be eaten earlier in the meal. In this country, the salad is either served before the entree or with it.

Commercially grown lettuce has been doused with insecticides and perhaps preservatives to keep it from wilting. These chemicals don't wash off easily—in many instances they are oily and not affected by water.

Vitamin A is found in lettuce, and vitamin C—which washes down the drain when you try to wash off the insecticide. Lettuce also has an abundance of potassium, sodium, calcium, magnesium, iron, and folic acid.

Leaf lettuce has long, loose, dark green leaves. They often have rust-colored crimped edges.

Bib lettuce, sometimes called Boston lettuce, is shaped like a green rose. The leaves are mild in flavor and tender, and cupping like a rose, make pretty salads.

Iceberg lettuce is a compact head of lettuce and is crisp but is lighter in color—not dark green to the core—and from the point of view of nutritionists not as valuable.

Salads became fashionable in the eighteenth century in France when an impoverished nobleman mixed a salad for a friend and was paid a fee for his services. Later, in London, he again performed the same service and his salads became the talk of London—he became a "gentleman salad maker."

Salads can be elegant and witty; they can be robust and hearty. They can be anything you want to make them—most salads these days are not very imaginative. A leaf of lettuce and a slice or two of undernourished, soggy tomato.

Mushrooms, like truffles, are fungi—not the kind of plants vegetables and grains are, but plants that also include rusts, molds, and mildews.

Fungi do not reproduce by seeds. They reproduce by spores. When a mature plant is laid on a white surface, the fine black dust you see is made up of spores. Not very appetizingly, the spore produces a stringy white substance called the *spawn* which penetrates dried manure or similar substances and eventually develops into a mushroom.

Since we're always looking for the source of vitamins, for instance, it's possible to speculate that since B vitamins are produced in the intestinal tract of animals, perhaps that accounts for the abundance of B vitamins in mushrooms.

Mushrooms are rich in folic acid. They keep company with brewer's yeast, raw wheat germ, soybeans, kidney, and liver. Vitamin B_{12} is a potent weapon against penicious anemia.

Mushrooms are also good sources of vitamin D, when they're grown in the sunlight. This vitamin doesn't occur in any other nonanimal source.

It's interesting that mushrooms contain no chlorophyll and yet are so nutritious. It's especially surprising to find that they contain vitamin D.

Mystery story fans, and most of us as children, know that some mushrooms are poisonous. "Amanita," the most poisonous of all, is one of the most beautiful growing things in the world. It is found in both America and Europe. Some are a soft, delicate green, while others are a flamboyant, flaming red spotted with white dots, or a cheerful orange, or a creamy off-white.

Mushrooms impart a flavor to almost any meal and are low in calories for those who are watching their weight.

The *pepper*, botanically speaking, belongs to the berry family. Peppers grow on plants that have shiny, dark green foliage. They can be eaten after they have attained any size, but actually, they are not ripe until they are red.

The pepper can be eaten raw, and should be—as often as possible—in salads or simply sliced and served with raw carrots, radishes, and celery.

Bell peppers are best known for their high vitamin C

content. The vitamin C increases as the pepper ripens, and in a fruit that is half green and half red, the vitamin C will be richer in the red section.

One ripe bell pepper may contain as much as three hundred milligrams of vitamin C; the average orange contains about fifty.

Pimentos and hot peppers are related to the bell pepper; all are high in vitamin C.

When vitamin C was first discovered, peppers were used as its only source. Many of the natural, vitamin C preparations are made from peppers, as well as from rose hips and other vitamin-rich sources.

Peppers contain vitamin A, three of the B vitamins (thiamin, riboflavin, niacin) as well as calcium, phosphorus and iron. They are also a source of vitamin P, which was first extracted from peppers, paprika, and citrus fruits.

Peppers are low in calories—they're considered a 5 percent vegetable. One medium pepper only contains twenty-five calories.

Potatoes Columbus is said to have discovered the potato on the West Indian island of Hispaniola. The word *potato* derives from the West Indian. Columbus described the natives as being "nourished" by a "root." He compared these roots with pears or small melons. "When they ripen," he wrote, "they are dug out as beets and radishes are with us." He went on to observe that they were dried in the sun and then ground into flour and made into bread which was then boiled.

Sir Walter Raleigh planted potatoes in his garden in 1584 and then he took sacks of them to Ireland, where they gained rapid popularity. The people of Ireland were extremely poor, and the potato will grow well even in poor soil.

Most varieties of potatoes are brown; there are some pink-skinned potatoes also. One of these was cultivated and eaten by the Incas, who lived in Chile and Peru. Reports are that we have "cultivated" some of our pink-skinned potatoes, too, by adding a highly toxic weed killer which intensifies the pink color.

Organically grown vegetables, or at least carefully grown vegetables must be insisted upon by the general public because consumer opinion determines the actions of the producer. If white celery and pink potatoes are favored by the public, the producer will oblige.

In the case of the potato, particularly, the skin contains many rich minerals and vitamins. To unknowingly, or from necessity, discard the skins deprives us of the most valuable portion of this vegetable.

While it is true that potatoes are 20 percent starch, they do contain a small amount of protein, and the quality of the protein is good. The essential amino acids are present in the potato. So don't classify potatoes with white bread. The latter is very nearly worthless as a nourishing food; potatoes are a "health food" when properly grown.

Pumpkins are a member of the gourd family and are not often used as a vegetable in this country. The Greeks knew them, and the word *pumpkin* comes from *pepon*, which means cooked in the sun. They are not, as one might think, native to this country.

Pumpkins are a natural food, prepared by nature—and, like the eggplant, have a thick, protective covering.

Pumpkins are particularly high in vitamin A.

Green, leafy vegetables For good nutrition, we are urged to eat green, leafy vegetables at least once a day. What are those green, leafy vegetables? Iceberg lettuce is the most commonly used and perhaps the least nutritious. It, like blanched celery, is almost white, and has a bland taste. The best greens are those that are very green, because they have more chlorophyll, minerals, and vitamins.

In general, leafy vegetables are rich in calcium and low in phosphorus. This makes them excellent additions to diets high in cereals, because there the balance is reversed.

Iron and potassium are available in good quantity from fresh, leafy vegetables. Parsley is very high in iron.

Romaine has a sharper taste than leaf lettuce. Its leaves are large, dark green, and spear shaped.

Endive is also called chicory. It has curly, lighter green leaves, with a mild to bitter taste.

Escarole is a broad-leafed endive, sharp in taste, deep green in color. It is usually chopped with other greens.

Watercress is a delicate green. Watercress sandwiches are enjoyed by some; others use watercress as a garnish, as the basis for a salad, or as a mixed green.

Tomatoes Summer tomatoes are superior to the hothouse variety and to winter tomatoes. Tomatoes tend to be pale and tasteless in the winter and spring, but fresh, juicy, and of a rosy color when picked from the vine on a hot summer day—these are highest in food value, too.

For the highest vitamin content, tomatoes should be ripened in bright sunlight and not picked until they are completely ripe. Ethylene gas is sometimes used to ripen commercially-grown tomatoes, which are picked green. The gas causes production of the bright-red tomato color. But tomatoes treated this way tend to be tasteless and nutritionally inferior.

Tomatoes are high in vitamins A and C.

FRUITS

There are literally hundreds of different kinds of fruits grown or gathered from plants, and many of these kinds have hundreds and sometimes thousands of varieties.

There have been several thousand varieties of apples developed in the United States alone. About twenty-five varieties form the bulk of the commercial crop, but there are one hundred varieties grown commercially.

Fruits can be divided into three classes, according to the climates in which they are grown.

The most important tropical fruits for export include bananas and pineapples. Hundreds of other kinds of tropical fruits are grown and eaten by those living in the tropics, but very few are marketed.

Subtropical fruits include members of the citrus group—oranges, tangerines, limes, grapefruit, and lemons. Other subtropical fruits include figs, dates, and olives. (The avocado can also be called a subtropical fruit, although it is less resistant to cold than the others.) Citrus fruits are simply large, pulpy berries, encased in thick, oil-bearing rinds.

Temperate zone fruits include a large number of commercial varieties. In terms of major production, probably the most important are grapes and apples. Other fruits in this group are pears, plums, peaches, and apricots, and such berries as strawberries, raspberries, blackberries, cranberries, blueberries, gooseberries, and currants.

Fruits are a very important part of our diet. They contain acids, salts, and vitamins that are needed for a balanced, healthy diet. They also make good laxatives because of the water and roughage they all supply.

All fruits contain one or more of the vitamins that are necessary to good health. They are especially good sources of vitamin C. Their sugar content makes them nourishing. Several minerals are found in fruit, including iron, phosphorus, and calcium.

The use of fruit as a part of man's diet, dates back to early civilizations. For thousands of years men have grown grapes, apples, pears, peaches, plums, dates, figs, olives, oranges, and lemons.

Interestingly enough, many of the berries have only been cultivated for several hundred years, including raspberries, blackberries, dewberries, strawberries, and cranberries. And blueberries for an even shorter time. But long before these plants were cultivated, man ate wild berries—those that grew where he was living. Many mentions of them are made in the writings of early civilizations.

As people migrated to different parts of Asia and Europe, they carried the seeds of fruit plants with them. Europe has had a dense population and good conditions for fruit growing. Europe produces more fruit than any other continent, with leading countries including Spain, France, Italy, and Greece. Predominant fruit crops of Europe are grapes, apples, pears, olives, and citrus fruits.

Asia produces a great quantity of fruit—but most of it is eaten in the countries where it is grown.

Australia, New Zealand, Argentina, Chile, and Brazil are also important fruit-producing countries.

Many fruits were brought to this country by Europeans as the New World was settled. Seeds were brought from the fruit-growing trees of Europe and planted here. But until about 1860 there was very little commerce in fruits. Fruits that were grown in a particular part of the country were eaten there.

Brought in from Asia and Europe were apples, pears, plums, cherries, quinces, figs, olives, dates, currants, gooseberries, and the Old World grape. Our oranges, lemons, and grapefruit originally came from Southeast Asia. Peaches, apricots, and Japanese plums came in from China and Japan.

The United States is the leading consumer and producer of fruits. Native to this country and developed here are the grapes of the eastern states—red and black raspberries, blackberries, dewberries, varieties of gooseberries, blueberries, cranberries, and native plums.

Fruits may be classified as pomes, drupes, nuts, or berries.

Pomes are core fruits, of which pears and apples are examples.

Drupes are stone fruits which include the cherry and the peach.

Nuts are considered dry-stone fruits, although the classification overlaps and they are also considered seeds. Almonds and walnuts are good examples of this.

Berries include the strawberry, and also the orange and grape. The blackberry is actually a cluster of drupes.

Apples are good for you. The natural sugars in apples are easily digested. Their sugar content is not as high as that in grapes, figs, dates, or prunes, for example.

The health-giving qualities of apples have been recognized for centuries, and apples have been prescribed by physicians. Yet, even today, scientists are not sure which ingredient is responsible for this characteristic. Is it the acid in the apple, the pectin? As with honey, we must believe that nature's combination defies scientific analysis in finding out just what it is in apples that is so good for the digestive tract.

Apples are low in calories and are a good reducing food.

Apples aid the body in absorbing iron from food. Also, the decalcifying effect of apples is less than that of any other food except carrots.

The sunny side of the apple contains more sugar and vitamin C than the shaded side; the skin contains more vitamin C than the pulp.

Apples vary in their vitamin C content. But all of them are a readily available source of this vitamin. Human beings, along with guinea pigs and monkeys, are the only creatures that do not manufacture their own vitamin C and we need it daily.

So a fresh, organically grown apple a day is good nourishment and good protection, too.

Bananas Alexander the Great found people in India eating bananas in the third century B.C.

This tropical fruit is nourishing and not so high in calories as is popularly supposed—only about eighty-eight to an average banana, and these are not "empty" calories—they're full of nutrients.

Bananas contain B vitamins, and are particularly high in vitamin A and also contain vitamin C.

Fully ripe bananas have dark specks in them; at this stage they are not rotten at all. In fact, the specks indicate the starch has changed into a completely digestible fruit sugar.

The banana has an alkaline reaction in the body, as do most fruits, and should be high on your list of healthful foods.

Cantaloupe As a source of vitamin C and vitamin A, the cantaloupe compares very favorably with the citrus fruits—without any of the citric or other acids.

A juicy, vine-ripened cantaloupe, picked in the height of the summer, is flavorful and nutritious. In the winter, cantaloupes tend to be rather tasteless although their vitamin content has not diminished. Cantaloupes taken from the vine and ripened artificially lack the flavor of vine-ripened ones because the sugar content increases as the melon matures naturally. When will we learn?

In addition to vitamins A and C and minerals such as calcium, phosphorus, iron, and copper, cantaloupe is high in one of the B vitamins—inositol—which is also found in peanuts, peas, beef brain and heart, and raisins, as well as wheat germ and brewer's yeast.

Dates are an ancient and venerable food. It is generally thought that they were used in the Near East and India before the Bronze Age.

The date grows on the date palm, which may grow to eighty or one hundred feet in height. Date trees have a long harvesting season, lasting in Southern California from September into early January. The dates on a single tree do not all ripen at the same time and have to be picked as many as eight times in a season. Date palms need a warm climate and large amounts of water. Southern California is about the only place in the United States where date palms can be grown. Each tree produces from two hundred to three hundred and fifty pounds of dates in a year.

Dates have a high sugar content, and make a nourishing and satisfying dessert in place of empty calories. Their calories do count, however, and if you're reducing you'll need to count how many you've eaten. It's hard to stop.

The sugar content of the date, like the cantaloupe, increases as the dates ripen, and fully ripe dates may contain as much as 75 percent sugar. They're fairly rich in minerals and also contain some vitamin B and A.

The fig is one of those health foods like yogurt and honey that have been used for centuries. Pliny, the Roman naturalist, wrote about them.

They probably originated in South Arabia; the Greeks knew about them and the Romans planted them in England. The Bible mentions them frequently, and, as with honey, they were used medicinally—as a curative—and for the maintainance of good health.

Figs are probably most noted for their effectiveness as a laxative. It is probably the bulk fiber and seeds of the fig that are responsible, although it may be the acids and minerals.

The fig contains a protein-dissolving enzyme called fictin. It is similar to the enzymes both in papaya and pineapple. Interestingly enough, this enzyme could be used to tenderize meat.

On the island of Majorca, not rennet or lactic acid, but fig branches are used to curdle milk. The enzyme in figs apparently acts in the same way on the casein (the protein) in milk, causing it to separate from the whey.

Figs have a high mineral content—much higher than most other foods. Only nuts and one or two cheeses have a higher calcium content. Figs are also richer in iron and copper than most fruits. To buy raw figs, generally you must be in an area where they are grown locally. Figs are highly perishable and shipping presents difficulties. Mediterranean countries distil figs and make them into a wine. We originated the "fig newton"—a cookie containing figs which was made in the town of Newton, Massachusetts.

The peach was first cultivated in China. Ancient caravans carried peach trees to Persia where Alexander the Great found them and carried them with him back to Europe. It was Spanish ships that carried peaches to the New World, and it was Spanish monks who planted peach trees around missions in the American Southwest. Today, they are grown on trees all over the country, in northern as well as southern sections.

The skin of the peach contains more vitamins than the rest of it. Organically grown peaches should be eaten, skin and all. Just be sure you defuzz it.

Peaches have an alkaline reaction in the digestive system, even though they contain three of the fruit acids—malic, tartaric, and citric.

Peaches, aside from their delicious, refreshing flavor, are most valuable for their vitamin A and C content.

Pineapples were used in early America as a symbol of hospitality. They're found carved and painted on colonial furniture.

In the winter and spring, when there are not many vitamin C—rich foods, the pineapple is available. Like other fruits, the vitamin C content of pineapples differs, depending on when they are picked and the way in which they are grown. Being a tropical fruit that is shipped to this country, they are picked greener than they would be if grown locally.

Pineapple, like the papaya and the fig, contains a protein-digestive enzyme. Papaya enzyme is sold commercially as a meat tenderizer. A fruit cocktail of fresh pineapple is good for digestion of your meat course.

Canning methods are generally good in Hawaii. The fruit is picked ripe and is usually in the can within thirty-six hours.

There would seem to be little excuse for poor canning methods, would there? Except those that economics create. For the consumer to insist upon the impossible is foolish, but for him to demand the possible is a responsibility we all have in the interest of our own and others' good health. When a process is healthful but uneconomical, there's going to be a conflict.

The skin of the pineapple is protection for the fruit against poisonous insecticides; it's not edible—being too spiny and tough.

When you're buying a pineapple, usually the heavier it is, the better the quality of the fruit. The fruit should be a dark, orange-yellow color and should smell fragrant. The "eyes" should be flat, almost hollow.

A pineapple is about 12 percent sugar, and is satisfying and healthful as a dessert.

A well-grown pineapple gives you vitamin C, vitamin A, a

small amount of vitamin E, several of the B vitamins, and various minerals.

Prunes are perhaps best known for their laxative qualities. We don't know exactly why, except that they have a high cellulose content.

Prunes are made from plums. They come originally from the Caucasus and the Caspian Sea. Then they were brought to central Europe and the Balkans. Today they're grown mostly in California.

Prunes drop to the ground and are harvested. The tiny cracks are formed when they are dipped in a milk alkaline solution to boil. This is how the drying process is done. The moisture escapes evenly. Some prunes are still sun dried, but the dehydrating process is more usual today. Avoid prunes that have been dried with sulphur.

Prunes are sorted and packed according to size. The label will tell you. There can be as many as eighty-five small ones to a pound; large ones may run under forty.

Prunes produce an acid reaction in the body, unlike other fruits which are alkaline in effect (excluding plums and cranberries). If enough other fruits and vegetables are eaten, the acidity of the prunes helps the acid-alkali balance in the system.

Prunes contain very little vitamin C. They are high in vitamin A and minerals, especially iron. They are also a good source of some of the B vitamins, including thiamin, riboflavin, niacin and pantothenic acid.

Watermelons have an interesting history. They were known, along with other melons, to the Greeks and Romans, who recognized their health-giving properties. Then, for some reason, people stopped eating melons, and it wasn't until translators of Greek and Roman texts came upon the word that an investigation was made of these vegetable fruits.

Watermelons, so much a part of "Americana," were first

brought here in the seventeenth century by the English.

Watermelons are a favorite summer fruit; they're cool and refreshing. They have pure water distilled by nature, natural sugar, vitamins, and minerals.

The thick rind of the watermelon protects it from poisonous sprays. Watermelon is a natural food and a healthful one.

Watermelon seeds are also nutritional. The Cuban Queen variety, which is really a gigantic member of the cucumber family, is very high in linoleic acid, one of the essential fatty acids contained in the oil of seeds.

SEEDS

The seed is the source of life; it probably contains the best balance of nutrients in nature.

The seed is the means of survival of the species. Many scientists think that because of this, its composition doesn't vary as widely as that of other foods.

The seed not only is the life source—it sustains it. All seeds contain vitamin B_1 —because this vitamin is necessary before seeds can sprout.

Seeds contain vitamin E. They contain unsaturated fatty acids; they contain minerals and proteins.

The catagory of seeds includes, in addition to such seeds as sunflower and sesame, all nuts, grains, beans, peas, soybeans, and lentils.

Seeds and leaves complement each other.

The mineral that abounds in seeds is phosphorus. From the point of view of nutrition and health, it is an important mineral. Leaves and grasses are low in phosphorus. Feed for horses and cattle should include phosphorus.

We get phosphorus in cereals, legumes, nuts.

Foods that are high in vitamins (like fresh fruits and salads) don't have as much phosphorus in them. Compared to a pound of lentils or beans, wheat or oats, you would have to eat a bushel of apples or a bushel of oranges for the same amount of phosphorus—or eleven pounds of beets or nine and one-half pounds of carrots.

Phosphorus is present in all the cells of the body. In

the quantity of minerals present in the body, calcium is first and phosphorus second. The two minerals are interrelated, and it's not so much the amount present as the ratio between the two. It should be two and one-half to one, with calcium predominating.

A diet chiefly of fruits and vegetables is apt to be lacking in phosphorous. Meats, cereals, and nuts improve the balance.

Living chiefly on cereals causes a more serious problem. Cereals have very little calcium and what little they do have is destroyed during the refining process.

In addition, the phosphorus that cereals do contain is in a chemical combination called phytate which combines with calcium whenever it can. So additional calcium is lost. Plenty of calcium-rich foods should be eaten: milk, yogurt, fruits, vegetables, green, leafy vegetables.

What about seeds needing other foods to complement them? Your body doesn't use phosphorus unless there is calcium present. If you're eating a lot of seeds—cereals, nuts, legumes—be sure you're getting calcium, too.

Bone meal is a good supplement. It contains the right combination of phosphorus and calcium.

In addition to phosphorus, seeds are rich in iron. The iron is removed from cereals in the milling process as the iron is removed from sugar cane and left in the blackstrap molasses.

The seed, wheat germ, is rich in iron. So are other seeds. So when we refine cereals, we remove the calcium, the iron and the B vitamins.

Magnesium is another mineral in which seed foods are rich: almonds, barley, lima beans, Brazil nuts, cashew nuts, corn, whole-wheat flour, hazelnuts, oatmeal, peanuts, peas, pecans, brown rice, soy flour, walnuts.

What about vitamins in seeds? The most important content is B vitamins and vitamin E. Seeds seem to need them, as we do, to grow. The B vitamins are important for the health of the nerves. It is tempting to draw conclusions about the general up-tightness of much of the population and the lack of B vitamins in most diets.

The B vitamins are necessary for the digestive tract. A great many television commercials offer relief for various digestive problems.

Vitamin E is necessary for the reproductive processes. It's important for the health of every muscle in the body. Refining foods has removed vitamin E; therefore, nutritionists are now helping us find other sources. Bread should be the staff of life.

Vitamin F, which is not as well known as some of the other vitamins, is plentiful in seeds. It is unsaturated fatty acids. Also, the essential lecithin is found in seeds. Lecithin keeps cholesterol in emulsion so that it doesn't collect in unwanted ways in the body.

The most important elements in seeds as foods, then, are their mineral vitamin, and protein contents. As for minerals (and remember, these are mostly lacking in refined foods like processed cereals and white bread), the most important are phosphorus and iron. Also remember that if you eat large amounts of seed foods, you should include calcium-rich foods in your diet also—green, leafy vegetables and fruits. Bone meal is good, also.

Considering the vitamin content of seeds, we find the B complex, vitamin E, and also unsaturated fatty acids and lecithin. Eat seed foods fresh, unrefined, un-tampered with.

There is also protein in these foods. There is a controversy between vegetarians and those who are not. Vegetarians believe that they can get sufficient protein in fruits, vegetables, nuts, and cereals. The question revolves, from a nutritional standpoint, around the completeness of vegetable versus animal proteins. We are made chiefly of protein—nails, hair, skin, bones, body fluid. The building blocks of protein are amino acids. The body rearranges them and uses them in the forms that it needs.

Of the vegetable proteins, corn is so lacking in the amino acid tryptophane that a diet where corn is the only protein will cause disease.

Peanut flour is high in most of the amino acids. But it is too low in methionine and tryptophane to be considered a complete protein.

Soybean flour which is probably the nearest to having complete proteins, is also considered a little low in methionine and tryptophane. If you are a vegetarian, and use soybean flour as your source of protein, you should also eat other foods rich in methionine and tryptophane at the same meal.

A vegetarian who eats eggs will not have this problem. The vegetarian who takes brewer's yeast will be getting complete proteins. The worn-out protein cells of the body must be rebuilt.

Seeds will not form a healthful diet by themselves, but as a supplement they are excellent. Nutritionists feel that more protein is needed daily than most people get. Seventy grams for an adult man; 60 for the average woman; from 40 to 100 grams for children, depending on their age and activity.

Incomplete proteins, when eaten with other foods that contain complete proteins, are used by the body.

Candy or soda?—try nuts or sunflower seeds.

Did you know that the seed of an Indian lotus plant was buried for over two hundred years and then sprouted? Or that melon seeds can sprout after thirty years? What is it in these seeds that is so vital, so resistant to time? The B vitamins and the sex and fertility vitamin—vitamin E.

The nutritive substance in seeds in concentrated, so concentrated that the root, stem, and several leaves are formed from the seed itself. No food is needed from the soil.

The seed is not as affected by the use of chemicals as are leaves or stalks. In one experiment, a chemical fertilizer was used on alfalfa. The inorganic phosphorus of the fertilizer went to the stalks and leaves, while the seed rejected the inorganic phosphorus.

Unsaturated fatty acids are obtained chiefly from seeds. Many seeds have an old and fascinating history.

Acorns are commonly associated with the American Indian. But there are oak trees in other parts of the world, too. Contemporary man eats them in Spain, Portugal, and Italy as we here, today, eat chestnuts. Acorns have a high oil and starch content; they're nutritious, and foods made from them are easily digestible.

Aniseeds Anise derives from the Greek *aneson*. These are a plant of the carrot family. The Romans ate aniseed cakes to aid digestion. A liqueur is made from anise seeds called anisette.

Apple seed oil is rich in vitamin E.

Banana seeds There aren't any. In its wild state, the banana was almost filled from one end to the other with large seeds that were like stone, with just enough pulp to attract birds and wild animals.

Barley is a cereal. In some parts of the world it is used for bread making. In this country it is used chiefly to make beer. Fermented barley makes malt which is used to make beer. Barley is perhaps the oldest cereal food. It was cultivated in China twenty centuries before Christ, and was known in ancient Egypt, Greece, Rome, and in ancient Switzerland among the lake dwellers.

Basil (a herb) is a fragrant plant of the mint family.

Berries Strawberries have many seeds. They're not particularly rich in sugar; they have a mild stimulating effect on digestion.

Buckwheat is not generally used in this country. New York State and Pennsylvania produce it. Buckwheat cakes are familiar, particularly on the eastern seaboard. Freshly ground buckwheat flour is excellent. Most of it sold commercially is refined, with other refined flours added. Buckwheat has a distinctive flavor. Many farmers plant buckwheat for its honey. Buckwheat honey has a distinctive flavor; it's dark in color and therefore richer in vitamins and minerals.

Caraway seeds were known to the Egyptian priest-physician before the book of Exodus was written. Caraway is used in rye bread, applesauce, soups, and stews.

Cardamom is an oriental herb, used in cakes and cookies. Its seeds have a pleasant, aromatic odor and a spicy taste. In the Orient they are chewed, like betel nuts.

Carob seed pods Carob trees are related to the honey locust tree. We don't eat the seeds of the carob fruit—we eat the pods. These are the fruits of the tree and are also called St. John's bread. This may be the food spoken of in the Bible as "locust." Carob has gained popularity as a chocolate substitute. It's sweet and has a chocolatelike taste. It's rich in proteins, carbohydrates, vitamins, and minerals.

Celery seed is good for seasoning soups, stews, and salads, if you like the taste of celery.

Coconut The classification here varies—all the coconut inside the outer shell is a seed, the largest of the seeds. Coconut palms grow on beaches near the sea, and their seeds are rich in nutrients. Eat the brown skin that encloses the white meat—many of the minerals and vitamins are here. In tropical countries, coconuts form the main staple of the diet and are considered a particularly nutritious food.

Corlander seeds The ancient Chinese thought that these seeds confer immortality. If that idea appeals to you, crush them and use them in cakes, bread, sausage, or cheeses. The food industry uses them to make gin and curry powder.

Corn is America's most famous grain (seed).

Cucumber seeds are mentioned in old English writings. They were used for medicinal purposes to help coughs.

Cumin seed is a spicy seed and was extremely common during the Middle Ages. It contains tannin and is one ingredient of curry powder.

Dill seeds in the East, are ground and eaten as a condiment. It's an old herb; it was sometimes chewed in church by the early settlers of this country. The reason is obscure. Dill oil, along with corlander seeds, is used in the manufacture of gin. Dill adds zest as a flavoring for soups, salads—anywhere you might enjoy the dill flavor.

Elderberry seeds are used for making elderberry wine and elderberry jelly: both are excellent.

Fennel seeds come from a tall herb of the carrot family; these seeds are very aromatic and are used in cooking.

Fig seeds are very small and are one of the few seeds that are eaten with fruit. They should be chewed; they are nutritive.

Flaxseed is best known for its use in making linseed oil. In Eastern Europe, it is used as a cooking oil. There's a nice legend about the flaxseed—gather them by the full moon and they make good love potions. From the sublime to the practical, they're a good source of unsaturated fatty acids. They've been used in other civilizations; the Greeks and Romans ate them like nuts.

Hempseed we associate with hemp and the manufacture of rope. These seeds are eaten in India and are preferred to sesame seeds. Hashish, the drug, is made from hemp leaves and resin.

Lentils, what are lentils? They're a plant of the pea family, and their seeds are small and edible. It's possible that they're the oldest cultivated vegetable. All ancient peoples seemed familiar with them; references are made to them in mythology. If you're in a church in Italy on Ash Wednesday, you'll see them planted in earthen pots. This is part of an ancient rite still observed, dating back to the days when Christians were worshipping down in the catacombs outside Rome. They wanted flowers but none would grow without light. But they discovered both wheat and lentils would sprout and grow in the dark. So, lentils were planted on Ash Wednesday and carried to the altar on Maundy Thursday.

Lentils are nutritious; use them in any recipe that calls for dried beans. They go well with garden vegetables such as tomatoes, and onions and mix well with vinegar, mustard or mushrooms.

Lettuce seeds There are such things; used in the Middle Ages, they were mixed in a plaster and used to induce sleep.

Lotus seeds have traditionally been eaten by Eastern peoples. Nutritionally, they are rich and protein and minerals—calcium, phosphorus and iron.

Their yellow or purple flowers are famous and exotic; the plant is an elegant member of the pea family.

Millet is a cereal which probably originated in Egypt.

The word millet today refers to any number of related cereals. It is used in the form of groats; it makes excellent bread, especially when used with wheat.

Millet is becoming popular in this country; it is used extensively in the East and is easily grown. Millet grass is used for hay.

Nasturtium seeds can be pickled if you wish, or you can use the leaves and seeds in salads. Nasturtium seeds are sometimes called Indian cress.

Nutmeg is a delightful spice. Mace is a part of the nutmeg seed. Both are used in cakes and cookies.

Okra seeds as a coffee substitute? This is a good brew.

The seeds are high in food value and very high in oil.

Parsley seeds are an old herbal remedy and with reason. The seeds are extremely high in vitamins A and C.

Pepper is a berrylike seed. It grows in hot, humid climates. You get white or black pepper depending upon how it is cured.

Pepper was once so highly priced that it became a medium of exchange. The Middle Ages used a great many spices—for preservatives as well as for perfumes.

Pine nuts There are many species of pine trees in this country, many of them containing edible nuts in their cones. Some are rich in starch, others in oil.

American Indians eat the pine nut. They grow wild; thus, are not chemically fertilized or chemically sprayed.

The *pinon* is another type of pine nut. They also grow wild and are not chemically treated.

Poppy seeds are of Oriental origin. Opium is made from the pods of the poppy; the seeds are used on breads and cookies.

Rye seed is another ancient cereal. It has been found in tombs dating from the Bronze Age.

The *sesame* is an East Indian plant whose edible seeds yield an oil. Their use reflects the wisdom of the ancients. They were one of the earliest seed crops cultivated by man. The sesame seed is mentioned frequently in Eastern legends. Halvah, a Turkish candy, is made from them.

Sesame seeds are extremely high in calcium. This is unlike most seed foods, which are low in calcium and high in phosphorus.

Sesame seeds are high in protein—higher than many meats. Of all the seed foods, including soybeans, they contain a higher proportion of the amino acids and are particularly rich in three of them.

They contain lecithin, which contains the unsaturated fatty acids. They contain B vitamins. Sesame is rich in inositol and choline, and also niacin. They are a good source of vitamin E. The oil made from the sesame is used as a cooking and salad oil and is rich in these nutrients.

Sesame goes well with honey, figs, dates, ground coconuts or broiled fish.

Sunflower seeds were once counted among the variety of seeds that we generally do not use, but which American Indians find very useful, among them juniper, salt-bush, tarweed, and wild sage. However, the sunflower is becoming more and more widely used. Most of the foods that were used by the Indians in their natural state have been tampered with, but the sunflower is a nutritious, natural food.

The Hopi depended upon sunflower seeds for flour and oil and ate the seed itself for nourishment. They used the stalks of the plant as fuel for fires; the ashes of these fires were then used as fertilizer for future crops—their method of organic gardening.

The sunflower itself resembles a daisy. The flower is sometimes sixteen inches in diameter, with one or two to a stalk. The flat face of the flower is actually a mosiac of round seeds.

What is the nutritional value of these seeds? The U. S. Department of Agriculture rates their protein as higher than all other vegetable plants; they also contain calcium, phosphorus, iron, vitamin A, nitrogen, thiamin, riboflavin, niacin and vitamin E.

The oil of sunflower seeds is important. The unsaturated fatty acids are necessary to health; commercial processing changes them into hydrogenated fatty acids or destroys them.

The B vitamins contained in the sunflower seed are considered one of the most important food elements for modern man.

SPROUTS

Sprouts contain more nutritional value than the seed from which they sprout.

In the Far East, sprouts are used as often as we use onions or celery.

The sprouted seed contains more vitamins than the seed.

Vitamin C increases as sprouted seeds grow.

Protein is manufactured in large amounts as the seed sprouts.

Sprouting is a new idea in this country; an old idea in those countries whose resources have been poor.

Soybean sprouts are rich in protein and fat, minerals—including calcium and iron—and vitamins.

What sprouts do we use?

Sprouts from almost every bean (especially the mung and soya).

Sprouts from peas.

Sprouts from lentils.

Sprouts from wheat.

Sprouts from alfalfa.

Sprouts from rye.

Sprouts from corn.

Sprouts from millet.

HONEY

Nature has supplied us with an assortment of natural sugars and honey is one of them.

Honey is a thick, sweet syrupy substance that bees create from the nectar of flowers. Some foods contain simple sugars, some double and multiple ones. Honey contains simple sugars. These sugars are absorbed quickly, while the others have to be digested.

The use of honey dates back to ancient times. The word honey is derived from the Arabic *han*. This became *honig* in German and *hunig* in Old English. Early Phoenician traders found so much honey being eaten in Britain that they named England the Isle of Honey.

English writers attribute much of the robust good health of early Britons at least partly to their use of honey. Honey was the only sweetener in England until the Middle Ages. The very rich began to use sugar then. It, alike white bread, came to symbolize wealth and position.

Mead, an alcoholic liquor made of fermented honey, was widely used. The same type of brew, called by various other names, was popular in other parts of Europe and Asia.

Honey is praised by every ancient religious book, and the remarkable manufacturer of this food was a symbol for several civilizations as well as for our own state of Utah. The industry of the bee was praised in ancient Egypt—kings were symbolized under this emblem. Honey was rewarded to the worthy; the sting to those who were not. The bee was also the emblem of the ancient French Empire. The royal cloak and flag were embroidered with many raised bees in golden thread. The emblem still appears on French china.

In the United States, the State of Utah is known as the Beehive State and has for its seal, a beehive surrounded by flowers, with the single word, "Industry." The first Mormons took with them the deseret or honey bee.

Though it is considered a "natural" food, honey is not a natural product occurring in nature, since it is manufactured by the bee and not produced by instinct. When the worker bee is born, he is equipped with all the necessary characteristics for honey-making, but he has to be taught how to use them. The bee serves quite an apprenticeship before it is allowed away on its own to collect nectar.

Bees work on a system. They are selective in the flowers they choose. They make about a thousand trips from the hive to the flower bed to collect one ounce of nectar, which loses 50 percent in evaporation.

The nourishing value of honey is dependent upon many factors—rain, sun, the mineral content of the soil, and whether the plant is grown in humus or artificial fertilizer. The flavor of the honey, of course, depends upon the flowers from which the bees have gathered their nectar. We have clover honey, sage, apple, orange. Wild plants are a natural source and are probably safer, because we need to know if the bees collected nectar from blossoms that haven't been sprayed.

If you buy other than blossom honey, you're also apt to be buying honey that is not in its natural state. Sometimes bees are fed sugar and glucose during the winter. Usually, the darker the honey, the more minerals, vitamins and enzymes.

We need sugar for energy; for optimum health, it should be obtained from unrefined, natural sources. Honey in its natural state is ready for absorption into the system, and requires no work to render it into a heat-producing power.

Athletes use honey for energy. Sir Edmund Hillary, who

scaled Mount Everest, used it. The great Indian wrestler, the Tiger, ate a great deal of honey. Because of its high caloric value and the ease with which it passes into the blood, it is one of the best foods for hikers, campers and mountain climbers.

In addition to being an excellent source of energy, honey is also said to be a mild laxative, a natural diuretic, and a mild stimulant. It is also considered a "safe" food, because bacteria can't live in honey—if the plants haven't been sprayed with insecticides.

BLACKSTRAP MOLASSES

Molasses is a thick, dark syrup produced during the refining of sugar. It's derived from the Latin *mel*, meaning honey.

When the sugar cane is boiled down and the pure sugar is removed, blackstrap molasses is left.

One tablespoon of the remaining molasses has as much calcium as you would find in a glass of milk; as much iron as you would find in nine eggs.

Blackstrap molasses is about 50 percent natural sugar. The lighter types of molasses are higher in natural sugar content.

Blackstrap has a mild laxative effect. It offers energy from its sugar content and is also nutritional. Since it is a highly concentrated food, small amounts should be used.

WHEAT GERM

In her well-known mystery novel, *Murder Must Advertise*, Dorothy Sayers wrote: "By forcing the damn-fool public to pay twice over—once to have its food emasculated and once to have the vitality put back again—we keep the wheels of commerce turning and give employment to thousands."

In its natural state, wheat will keep alive for thousands of years. When the tombs of Pharaohs were opened, wheat was found in them; when it was planted, it germinated.

In its emasculated state, it does not keep indefinitely, is devitalized and if we wish to eat the vital part of the wheat, we must, in one form or another, eat the wheat germ.

Wheat is one of the oldest of the domesticated grasses. Man found early that wheat was a sustaining food. By grinding and firing it, the indigestible cellulose could be broken down and, unlike meat, it did not putrefy, and so could be stored for long periods.

A grain of wheat is composed of three main parts: the endosperm, the bran and the germ. About 85 percent is endosperm; about 13 percent is bran and some 2 percent is germ.

The endosperm consists mainly of starch. It also has a large store of reserve plant food which helps the grain to germinate and the seedling to sprout and develop.

A layer encloses the endosperm which is rich in protein and is separated from the rest of the grain during the milling process. It is called semolina.

The bran is the protective outer covering.

The germ or embryo is that part of the grain from which the plant springs, when the grain is planted.

About forty years ago, scientists discovered that bran was rich in vitamin B_1. However, the germ contains more than 50 percent of all the vitamins. It is the only part of the grain that contains vitamin A.

The germ is also the richest known source of vitamin E, called the "fertility vitamin." The germ, in addition, stores the B complex vitamins.

It wasn't until the 1920s that scientists discovered the existence of the nutritive factor now known as vitamin E. Rats fed on a diet of protein, cornstarch, lard, fat, yeast and a salt mixture matured normally but failed to reproduce.

Later, a potent alcohol was isolated from wheat germ oil. It was fed to unproductive rats and it was found that it contained the missing substance—which was then named vitamin E.

It was also labeled "alpha-tocopherol" from *tokos* meaning "child-birth," *phero* meaning "to bear" and the suffix "ol" to indicate that it was an alcohol.

Further investigation showed that vitamin E was found in fresh meat, milk, butter, various grains and fresh vegetables. But vitamin E is most abundant in wheat germ.

More than 100,000,000 pounds of wheat germ are extracted in this country and Canada, much of it being available to the public in various forms. Since bread is the main source of wheat germ for most people, the wheat germ that has been refined should be replaced in the diet for maximum health.

Always use freshly milled wheat germ. As soon as the grain is ground into flour, the oils which contain vitamin E combine with oxygen and become rancid. This destroys vitamin E. Get wheat germ vacuum packed if possible, and keep it tightly covered and refrigerated.

ALFALFA

Alfalfa is a plant of the pea family. It is commonly used for fodder, for pasture, and as a cover crop.

Lately it has become important as a food for people. We're eating the leaves, the stems and the seeds.

It has been discovered that alfalfa is very rich in minerals. Probably because its roots go deep into the soil, seeking out minerals there. It has roots that are from ten to twenty feet long.

Alfalfa doesn't have to be resown every year as corn does.

You can buy alfalfa in tablet form, as a food supplement, or as seeds or leaves to make tea with.

You're drinking vitamin A in your alfalfa tea; you're also drinking the same vitamin E that animals get when they eat alfalfa—it's considered their richest source. Also very rich in vitamin K, alfalfa has cured high blood pressure in animals and might well do the same for humans.

You can chew the stalk and leaves of alfalfa if you like—you'll know what the cow tastes when she's munching happily, anyway. If you don't happen to have a taste for it, take it in tablets, or make tea with the leaves and stalks.

Natural it is—and good for you.

BONE MEAL

Bone meal is available in health food stores as a food supplement. It consists of the bones of healthy cattle, ground finely into a flour. It's usually taken with milk or a little water.

It's an excellent source of calcium and of phosphorus and fluorine. Bone meal is said to aid in the reduction and prevention of dental cavities.

The eating of bones is instinctive with many animals and primitive man followed their example. With civilization, the practice was stopped and man lost a valuable source of calcium.

DESICCATED LIVER

Desiccated liver is liver that has been dried, with all the vital nutrients still retained.

The liver might be called the storage depot of the body. This is why it is rich in so many health-giving elements. Liver is rich in the B vitamins, especially vitamin B_{12}. It is also an excellent source of vitamins A, C, and D and the minerals iron, calcium, phosphorus and copper.

Because of the widespread vitamin B deficiency that the refining and processing of foods has caused, liver should be eaten frequently. If you can't eat liver at meals at least once a week, visit a health food store and try some desiccated liver.

BREWER'S YEAST

Yeast is a yellow, frothy substance consisting of minute fungi that cause fermentation.

It's used for two purposes—baking and brewing.

Yeast occurs in nature as plants and has been known since the times of the early Egyptians. The yeast plant stores large quantities of vitamins for its own use, much as do other fungi—the mold on cheeses, mushrooms.

Brewer's yeast is an excellent source of B vitamins.

It contains complete proteins; as the animal proteins are complete proteins. Yeast, however, is a very concentrated source.

Brewer's yeast differs from baker's yeast. The yeast plants use B vitamins as a source of food. In baker's yeast, the plants are still alive and if eaten raw will absorb whatever B vitamins it can find.

Brewer's yeast, on the other hand, has been made specifically for food. The growing of the yeast plants can be controlled in such a way that the growers can predict what the protein and vitamin content of the final product will be. This is because the yeast is grown on a food substance called a *wort*. In breweries, cereal grains and hops are the wort. Yeast can be grown in a few hours.

Yeast contains no fat, starch or sugar.

If any food could be said to be a reducing food, it is brewer's yeast: Its excellent protein is satisfying, it satisfies the appetite, it increases the basal metabolism, it gives you pep to work off unwanted pounds.

Brewer's yeast is available in tablet or powdered form. Mix it with fruit or vegetable juices or drink it in milk. Some brands have a more pleasant taste than others. Experiment.

FISH LIVER OILS

The theraputic value of cod-liver oil was first discovered in England, where it was used to cure rickets. But many hundreds of years ago, those living in northern countries such as Iceland and Norway managed to render the oil from the livers of the fish they caught. They knew that it was good for their children.

It was not until recently that we have understood why fish-liver oil is so important to health. It contains concentrated amounts of vitamins A and D. Sunshine and fish-liver oils are the best sources of vitamin D; it is important for absorption and utilization of calcium in the body.

Try cod-liver oil capsules or halibut-liver oil capsules.

ROSE HIPS

After the petals fall from roses, a fruit grows. Birds like this fruit, and while this is not always a reliable guide, in this case it is.

Northern European countries have eaten rose hips, as a source of vitamin C, for many years. They use rose hips syrup in soups and puddings as well as enjoying a beverage called rose hips tea.

The content of vitamin C in rose hips is from ten to one hundred times greater than that of any other food.

KELP

Seaweed. It was considered food fit for the gods in ancient China.

Who is eating it? And where? And why?

They're eating it in Japan. Some of it is ground into flour and made into noodles; some of it is sweet and used for cakes.

Other northern countries have used it, although not extensively. In South Wales, the national dish is laverbread, and contains seaweed. In Ireland, they have something called dulse which is a seaweed they call "sea lettuce." It is said to look like spinach and taste like oysters.

Seaweed is a plant that grows under the sea. It comes in three colors—green, brown, and red. Seaweed has neither roots, nor leaves, nor seeds, nor flowers.

Seaweed has a simple structure and it may well be the first form of life that appeared on this planet.

Kelp is one of the brown seaweeds. The most valuable thing about kelp is its minerals, as might be expected from a sea plant.

How good a source of minerals the kelp is depends upon how good a source of minerals the sea is. The same is true of land plants, which derive their minerals from the soil in which they grow.

Of the minerals, it is the trace minerals for which kelp is particularly valuable.

Trace minerals include iodine, copper, manganese, zinc and others. The body needs only small amounts, but it needs them. As our soil becomes more eroded, the trace minerals are being washed away. Commercial fertilizer does not contain trace minerals; thus, unless organic farming is practiced, none are being put back.

What happens to these trace minerals that are being washed from the land? They are washed into the ocean and some of them are absorbed by seaweed.

Of the trace minerals in kelp or seaweed, iodine can probably be considered the most important. There are parts of the country where there is no iodine in the soil. Iodized salt is widely used and was encouraged by health authorities in an attempt to alleviate this problem. Other than iodized salt, it is difficult to find a good source of iodine occurring in natural composition.

MEAT

Young owners of health food stores hope we will go back to eating as we did in "grandmother's day."

This is a market, says one young man. It has all that you find in other markets. But we sell nourishing food. I've learned to eat for nourishment, he says, and food tastes better.

Our grandmothers recognized the need for protein: thick, juicy steaks, plump chickens and turkeys, succulent pork roasts, crisp bacon and fresh eggs; tall glasses of milk. If granny glasses and long skirts, sideburns and long hair are a protest against Madison Avenue and the organization man, they are also nostalgia for some and a welcome change of trend.

The word protein comes from the Greek and means "of first importance." Protein occurs in all living matter. It's made up of twenty-two amino acids of which the body can manufacture most but not all. Some have to be preformed, preferably all together in a single food or in a combination of foods.

For vigor and health, it is generally agreed that we need a liberal quantity of good protein.

The bodies of animals, alike our own, are composed largely of proteins. Meat, fish and fowl, therefore, are excellent food sources. When proteins are eaten, the digestive juices in the body convert them into amino acids. The proteins in the different parts of the body differ and the different parts of the body select those which it needs.

Most of the 22 amino acids are needed in forming every tissue in the body. All but eight of these, however, can be made from the cells from fat or sugar, combined with the nitrogen that is freed from used protein. There are eight which the body cannot make.

It's not easy to be sure you're buying meats which contain the nutrients you need. If you can raise your own chickens, turkeys, cattle and pigs, that's fine. If you can't, you must find meat and poultry of the highest quality.

Animals should be fed on nitrogenous and mineral-containing food. When cattle are allowed to range, they instinctively choose the plants that are best for them.

Meat is graded according to conformation, finish and quality.

Conformation refers, as the word implies, to the shape of the animal and consequently the cut. Cuts should be shapely, with full muscles and a large percentage of meat as compared to bone.

Finish refers to quality, color and distribution of the fat. The best finish is a smooth, even covering of creamy white, flaky fat over most of the exterior; and liberal deposits between the large muscles and muscle fibres. This is called *marbling*.

Quality refers to the firmness and strength of the muscle fiber and connective tissue, since these affect the tenderness of the meat. Texture of meat is related to quality.

POULTRY

Poultry is available all year. It is an excellent protein.

Be sure that the poultry you buy has not been given stilbestrol. This is used to induce quick weight, and antibiotics are used to keep poultry alive in an unnatural environment. Besides being inhumane, it is not healthful. Residues are left in the poultry.

With a minimum of processing, poultry is considered necessary to the well-rounded diet, in addition to meats and fish.

Chicken has a slightly higher protein content than beef or veal and is considerably higher in protein than pork or lamb. The same is true for turkey. Duck is slightly lower in protein content.

Chicken, turkey and duck are rich in phosphorus and contain calcium and iron as well as a plentiful supply of B vitamins.

Health food stores are beginning to carry meats and poultry for those who wish to include them in their diets. These animals have been raised on organic feed and under humane conditions.

FISH

Fish gives you about the same amount of protein as meat and eggs. However, it's lacking in vitamin A, which is stored in the inedible liver.

It's a rich source of phosphorus—ocean fish and sea foods are excellent sources of iodine. Ocean fish absorb valuable minerals from the sea water.

Most of the fish caught in commercial fishing areas go to factories that clean and process them. They are prepared frozen, canned, dried or smoked.

Clams and oysters have their shells removed before processing.

Some fishing vessels carry their own processing equipment. However, most fishermen carry their catches into port for processing. Workers wash and clean part of the fish; then they send it to market as fresh fish.

Fish come from lakes, streams and oceans. Seafoods include clams, lobster, crabs, oyster, scallops and shrimp. Many of these sources are becoming increasingly polluted and concern continues to be expressed.

Fish are an excellent source of protein, and cheaper than other animal proteins. There are a number of reasons.

No one has to plant or harvest fish.

No one has to worry over the proper proportion of elements in their diet.

Fishermen need only a boat, and even weather is not the problem that it is to the farmer and cattleman.

Fish have not always been inexpensive. In the 18th century, there was no refrigeration in England, for example, and the price of fish was extremely high. Only recently as 1820 did they pack fish in ice in England in order to transport them.

In the 16th century, England established two fish days. This legislation was designed to stimulate ship building. People who ate meat on these days were heavily fined.

Salt became an important item of trade, because most of the fish was salted in order to preserve it.

Fish is a big industry in this country. The Boston pier handles some 300 million pounds of fish each year. Nevertheless, the average American only eats around 15 pounds of fish products each year. This compares with 100 pounds of white sugar per person. The large amount of sugar consumed does not come as such a surprise; this fact has been publicized more and more. But, it is a surprisingly small amount of fish.

What is healthful about healthy, uncontaminated fish? Fish is chiefly protein, as is meat. It contains the necessary amino acids which are also contained in chicken and beef.

Fish contain valuable minerals. They contain fluorine, which has caused some concern, but the general opinion seems to be that fluorine which has been assimilated by fish from water—that is, organic fluorine, is not harmful.

Fish contain relatively large amounts of calcium, copper, iron, magnesium, phosphorus, potassium, sodium and strontium. It's the high phosphorus content that has caused fish to be referred to as brain food.

Fishmeal, in a category with other feed for animals, is highly concentrated and a highly rich food. As might be expected, it's an excellent source of B vitamins, especially B^{12}.

NATURAL VEGETABLE OILS

The principal sources of essential fatty acids are natural vegetable oils.

So many vegetable fats are hydrogentated and animal fats contain so little unsaturated fatty acids that natural vegetable oils are one of the few dependable sources.

Vegetable oils, as sources of linoleic acid, are needed to decrease blood cholesterol. Lecithin, a substance which breaks cholesterol into tiny particles which can pass readily into the tissues, is made of fat, cholin, inositol and essential fatty acids. Linoleic acid is the most important of these acids.

Corn oil contains from 35 to 70 percent linoleic acid.

Soybean and cottonseed oils contain the same amount.

Safflower oil contains from 85 to 90 percent.

Buy cold-pressed, unhydrogenated vegetable oils from your health food store. Use them in salads and for cooking.

HERB TEAS

The use of herbs goes back many centuries, when they were used both medicinally and for meal-time beverages. Coffee and chocolate were unheard of—or were known only to the wealthy.

Before drugs, herbs were the only medicines known. Every housewife had a herb garden.

For asthma sufferers:

        mullein
        sweet marjoram

If you have a nervous headache:

aniseed	mugwort
camomile	rosemary
catnip	sage
lemon balm	sweet marjoram
lemon verbena	

As remedies for rheumatism:

        wintergreen leaves
        boneset
        celery

For indigestion:

aniseed	fennel seed
basil	peppermint
beebalm	sage
boneset	

As a good spring tonic:

        coltsfood

Or as a blood purifier:

camomile	ground ivy
celandine	red clover
elderblossoms	sage

Each herb has its own unmistakable fragrance which is always fresh, clean-smelling and refreshing.

Try using herb teas.

WINEMAKING

Wines can be made from the juice of almost every fruit and vegetable.

Extract the juice, lace it with honey, and add a yeast starter.

Try apple juice, honey and yeast. You'll have a thoroughly healthy beverage: Minerals and vitamins in the honey; B vitamins in yeast: Potassium, calcium, sulfur and other minerals, plus vitamin C, in the apples.

Rhubarb, elderberry and parsnip wines are popular. And many herbs make excellent wines with health-giving properties. Try balm wine, clary, coltsfoot or sloe.

POP WINES

Americans have never had an ordinary table wine. "Pop" wines may be giving us our first true *vin ordinaire*.

Pop is what the wine-industry is calling their new product. It's named both for popular and for soda-pop. They think it may be the era of pop wines for the Pepsi generation and the era of "Cold Duck"—a new dinner wine—for the coffee crowd.

Three new pop wines are called "I," "Love" and "You." "I" is a white wine with a lemon and lime flavor; "Love" is pink, with fruit flavoring; "You" is grape with a cola flavor.

"Zapple" has an apple flavor.

"Annie Green Springs" is a rose wine which sells in half-gallon bottles wrapped in brown, Kraft-paper labels.

The I, Love and You labels were designed by Allan Aldridge, who did many of the Beatles' album covers.

Skier's "Vin Glogg" is a 20 percent desert wine, laced with cinnamon, vanilla and other spices. You drink it hot—it's popular with the after-ski set.

"Spinada" is a fruit-flavored red wine which is based on Spain's "Sangria." This Spanish wine is really a pop wine—a cheap red wine with all sorts of fruits and flavors used.

Pop wines are designed to appeal to everybody over 21 and under 35. They're made from grapes that cost much less than those used in premium wines. And they're not aged—the crush this fall becomes the pop wine next spring.

The pop boom has begun as a west coast phenonomon. "Cold Duck" is already popular nationwide.

Cold Duck tastes like champagne but has a lower alcoholic content.

Cold Duck has been around a long time. It was not named by an imaginative ad man but comes from the German. Back in 1920, bartenders in Europe used to pour leftover wines into a few bottles. One of the mixtures happened to be champagne and red burgundy. In Germany, they called these leftovers *Kalte ende* or "cold ends." This drink became a fad with the "Lost Generation" of the 1920s in Europe. *Kalte ende* was changed somehow to *Kalte ente* which translates as "cold duck."

We didn't know about it in this country until two or three years ago, when wineries began to produce it. Either the mood of the country is right, or it has been good all along—for whatever reason, it may be the largest single seller of wines within the next ten years.

Cold Duck is made with two fermentations: one to turn the grape juice into wine and a second to produce the sparkle. If it's fermented the second time in the bottle instead of in the bulk, it costs more but tastes better.

Grapes are healthful, as are lemons and limes. Apples are rich in nutrients. Wine stimulates the appetite and aids digestion. Pop wines may be a new "health food."

YOGURT

Since Biblical times, yogurt has been used primarily as a food. It's a thick, semisolid food made from milk, fermented by a bacterium. These microbes that give yogurt its distinction were separated and named Bacillus Bulgaricus.

Yogurt is a famous Bulgarian milk product and was brought to North America by the Rosell Institute of La Trappe Monastery in Canada. It has also been used for centuries in countries from Turkey to Lapland and Iceland to China.

Yogurt can be made from either cow's milk or goat's milk. It has the consistency of custard and is a delicious food. It is also a superior nutritional product.

Yogurt is an excellent source of protein.

It is also an excellent source of calcium. Calcium can only be absorbed in an acid medium which the lactic acid in yogurt supplies.

Yogurt is high in vitamins—especially vitamins B^1 and B^2. It is also easily digested. After an hour in the digestive tract, only 31 percent of milk is digested; 91 percent of yogurt is digested in the same time.

Yogurt has another, rather unique feature. It is a "factory" of hard-working bacteria which produce B vitamins for future use. Its bacteria also break down milk sugar into lactic acid in the intestines, and harmful bacteria are unable to live in that acid medium.

A study was made at Columbia University which pointed out that when yogurt was eaten over a long period of time, no other bacteria were found in the stools except those from yogurt.

One difficulty with commercially prepared yogurt which contains too much highly sweetened fruit is that sugar stimulates the flow of alkaline digestive juices in the intestine, which prevents the effective absorption of calcium.

Available in health food stores are flavored yogurt such as vanilla, which contains natural vanilla and brown sugar.

You can make your own yogurt if you want to. The culture can be obtained from a health food store. It's added to warm milk and the acid formed changes the milk to a thick custard. It should then be chilled at once to stop the bacterial growth and keep it from becoming too sour.

CEREALS AND BREAD

Jack Armstrong was the all-Americam boy for a generation raised on Wheaties, the breakfast of champions.

These "health-building" breakfast cereals unfortunately contain nothing much except some sugar, and starch that is converted to sugar. Also present are some artificially added nutrients which are questionable in value.

The commercially prepared, dry cereals have been the subject of widespread advertising. We need a few heroes for the younger set who eat whole grain cereals for breakfast. Surfers? Film-makers? Young entrepreneurs of organic restaurants such as "The Steaming of the Stew" and organic merchants of markets such as "The Radiant Radish"?

"In" and "healthy" may be becoming synonomous.

There are 1-1/2 grams of protein in a half a cup of commercially prepared wheat flakes.

There are 24 grams of protein in a half a cup of wheat germ.

Corn is the leading cereal in the United States. *Oats* are second. More oats are used in breakfast cereals than any other grains.

Take the oat grain and remove the tough hull; the groat remains. Unlike wheat, when oats are milled the germ and the bran remain. Oatmeal is a whole grain, containing more of the nutritional value of the original grain than wheat flour.

There's a legend of a famous giant in Wales who ate oatcakes and buttermilk; oats are a staple fare in this part of the world.

136

Rice is a cereal. Almost half the population of the world uses it as their basic food.

Brown rice contains all the nutrients of the grain.

The original brown rice as it comes from the plant contains protein, starch, fat, minerals and vitamins. When it's milled to make white or polished rice, it loses 10 percent of the protein, 85 percent of the fat and 70 percent of the minerals. There is also a significant loss in vitamins.

Fifty years ago it was discovered that polished rice was causing beriberi; now we "enrich" it. Maybe in another fifty we'll be back to the natural grain again.

Rye contains carbohydrates, as do all grains, but it is a good source of protein as well. Wheat tends to be more fattening while rye apparently contributes to muscle strength.

You can buy a cream of rye cereal at your health food store.

Millet is available as a cooked cereal; it offers some protein and other valuable nutrients. It's not as widely used, but is becoming more popular.

Bread should be made from whole-grain, stone-ground flour. It should be free from preservatives and should be kept refrigerated.

The art of bread-making has been largely lost in our busy, urban way of life. There are signs of a revival, however, of this most ancient of arts.

VITAMIN SUPPLEMENTS

If we could get all the nutrients we need from the foods that we eat, vitamin supplements wouldn't be necessary. Since this isn't always possible, we can supplement our diets with single vitamins or vitamins in combination.

Vitamins derived from natural sources are preferable to those that are synthetically made. There's a wide choice of vitamins available today. The labels contain information concerning the source of the product, whether natural or not, and from what food source; how much of the vitamin the product contains; and the minimum daily requirement of the vitamin if it is known (if it is not known, it will state that no minimum daily requirement is established or that the need in human nutrition has not been established).

Vitamin A, for example, is available in capsules derived from fish liver oils; tablets containing palmitate with lemon from grass oil; fast disintegrating tablets made only from palmitate. Capsules and tablets can be purchased containing 25,000 U.S.P. Units of Vitamin A; both are also available which contain 50,000 units of the vitamin.

Capsules and tablets containing both vitamin A and vitamin D are available and also a tablet containing A, D, and E.

Alfalfa tablets made from the green leaves of alfalfa can be purchased. Each tablet is equivalent to approximately four grams of fresh alfalfa leaves. You're on your own here—no minimum daily requirement has been established.

The B vitamins are available as single vitamins. Most

nutritionists feel, however, that only the B complex should be taken. When the B vitamins were first being discovered and the health-giving properties of each were reported, it was not realized that taking too much of one could cause deficiencies in the others.

B complex vitamins are available which are made from various natural sources. Some are in a natural yeast base with iron; some contain rice bran but no yeast or wheat products; others are made from brewer's yeast.

Bone meal tablets with vitamin D are available. One label notes that the bone meal is of the highest quality, derived only from selected bones of government inspected cattle.

Vitamin C is a well-known vitamin; not as well known are the sources other than citrus fruits that it can be derived from.

You can buy, for example, acerola C tablets. These include rutin, citrus bioflavonoids, acerola, rose hips, and green pepper extracts. There's available a lemon bioflavonoid complex, and a tablet called Honey Bee C tablets with Rose Hips. There are also the standard vitamin C tablets containing various amounts of the vitamin.

Vitamin D is available in fish liver oil capsules and capsules.

Vitamin E can be purchased as tablets or capsules. They contain International Units of from 100 to 400, depending on how much you wish to take. Usually these are made from vegetable oils.

There are also mineral supplements available and a good assortment of protein supplements. Of the proteins, some are made from vegetable sources and some from animal sources. You can buy an all vegetable protein supplement with a nut-like flavor made from wheat gluten and soy beans. Or you can buy an animal-vegetable supplement derived from casein, lactalbumin and egg yolk powder combined with soy bean extracts.

Read the labels and choose which seem right for you.

SOYBEANS

In areas where civilizations have flourished, it has been because man has found foods basic to his existence. The soybean is such a food. It has been used for centuries in Asia and it is possible that China survived as a nation because of this plant. Both nutritionally and as a medium of exchange, the soybean has been vital to the life of the Chinese.

Soybeans became a vital food in this country during the Second World War. They had been grown here for over a hundred years but were used as feed for animals. As a war emergency, however, they became an animal replacement food and have been important in our economy ever since.

Soybeans are a superior source of proteins. Some nutritionists rank them as one of the five major protein foods, along with meat, milk, fish and eggs. The beans are rather unique in their nutritional value because of their high percentage of protein and oil.

They are probably the best source of protein from vegetables and have been called "the meat that grows on vines."

They're low in carbohydrates, unlike other dry beans.

They contain both vitamins and minerals and are especially rish in calcium, phosphorus and iron.

There is a difference between green and dry soybeans. When soybeans are almost full size, but still green, they are considered a green vegetable. These green beans contain vitamin A, and B^1 vitamins and some vitamin C. They have a nut-like flavor and may be eaten as a vegetable themselves or may be mixed with other vegetables. Green soybeans can be purchased canned or frozen, or in packages ready to cook.

Dry soybeans are the mature beans removed from the pod. They differ in color, turning yellowish or gray-green in color. The dry beans are far richer in B vitamins than are the green beans; they contain less vitamin A, however, and no vitamin C.

Seasonings such as tomatoes or onions improve the rather flat flavor of these beans.

Roasted soybeans are popular. They're sometimes called salted or toasted soybeans. They're usually deep-fat fried and then salted. They should be kept in an airtight container.

Soybean oil is one of the more concentrated sources of unsaturated fatty acids. In addition, it contains vitamins A and D and is a good source of E and K.

Sprouted soybeans contain all the vitamin B complex of the bean plus a rich supply of vitamin C.

Soy milk has been made in China for centuries. You take the dry beans, soak and grind them, add water and then strain off after cooking. The milk ordinarily has a strong bean flavor. Soy milk is available now which has had this taste and odor removed. It now tastes sweet and rather nut-like. You might enjoy trying some. It can be bought in single-strength liquid and liquid concentrate, or it may be purchased in powder form.

Tofu, or soy cheese, is more commonly known in the Orient as bean curd. It's a soft, custardy white cheese with an unusual flavor. It has many uses in the menu: it can be used as we use cheese, or can be a meat or fish substitute or, properly seasoned, as a desert.

Soy flour has a variety of uses. The flour, surprisingly enough, is a product of the western world. While the Chinese have used stone mills to grind grains, they have never made soybean flour.

It is not a true flour in the sense that wheat and rye flours are, but it is a highly concentrated vegetable protein food. It is similar in food value to dry powdered milk.

Soy flour is a rich source of protein and of the B vitamin complex. It has a high content of calcium, phosphorus and potassium, as well as liberal supplies of copper, magnesium and iron.

It is almost starch-free and has an alkaline reaction in the body. You can buy either full-fat or low-fat soybean flour. The full fat contains up to 20 percent fat, and a high protein content of 40 to 50 percent. Low-fat flour has most of the fat removed.

Soy flour is being used as a natural additive in several kinds of foods. Some candy makers are using it as an emulsifier; it is also being used in baked goods. The meat industry is taking advantage of its high protein value and adding it to meat loaves and meat preparations.

Soy bread is also made from soy flour. Since it contains no gluten or starch to bind it, it must be mixed with other flours.

Soybeans have been made into coffee substitutes. The liquid looks like coffee but has a different aroma and flavor.

Soy sauce has long been known to Americans as an Oriental flavoring. The sauce is made from whole beans, and the dark color occurs during the processing.

The soybean has reason to be called the "king of the legumes."

RAW JUICES

It is not really understood why fresh fruits and vegetables are so good for health. It is not only their vitamin and mineral content. But we do know that they play a part in not only maintaining but restoring good health.

Raw juices are particularly recommended for their theraputic value.

Our bodies need a chemical balance. Too little calcium causes deficiencies in the teeth and bones. The calcium-phosphorous balance, if not correct, can cause nervousness.

Nature offers vital nutrients in the correct balance for health. In reproducing substances, biochemists can only use those substances they know about.

The cellulose of vegetables is valuable, but the potency is increased in juices. Some nutritionists feel that the use of fresh raw juices will rejuvenate the system.

Try drinking fruit and vegetable juices every day—they give you natural stimulation rather than the artificial stimulation of tea or coffee.

Natural juices have been used for a long time as nature's remedies for various ailments. Nature will cure when given a chance; nature will offer excellent health building nutrients when they are used in their natural state.

Commercially prepared juices are often diluted with water and artificially sweetened. In addition to additives and preservatives. To be healthy, drink pure fresh juices.

There's a difference between a juicer or liquifier and a blender. The blender purees food, whereas the juicer or liquifier removes the fiber, leaving the pure juice.

The fruits and vegetables you choose should be tender and young, solid and with a deep color. Don't be tempted to use wilted foods, just because they're going to be ground up.

Fruit juices are thought to preserve and increase the alkaline reserve in the blood stream. Fruits are usually divided into three groups: acid, sub-acid and sweet fruits. The main fruit acids are malic, tartaric, citric and oxalic. Malic acid is found in such fruits as apples, grapes, berries, pineapples and cherries. Tartaric is found in limes, lemons, grapefruit, oranges—imparting a tart flavor. Oxalic acid is in small amounts in such fruits as raspberries, grapes, and tomatoes. A very small amount is found in oranges, lemons and apples.

Alkaline elements, which are combined with these acids, give most fruits their alkaline reaction.

Apple juice is rich in magnesium, iron, silicon and potassium. Apples also contain the beneficial mallic acid. Apple juice is especially rich in vitamin C.

Orange juice is an excellent source of vitamin C.

Pineapple juice contains a good supply of vitamins and minerals in addition to its digestive factors.

Grape juice is considered particularly healthful. Those who take the "grape-cure" in health resorts in Europe live on grapes exclusively for a month to six weeks, eating as much as eight pounds of grapes daily. The cure is said to be particularly helpful with respiratory problems and anaemic conditions.

Carrot juice is one of the most valuable vegetable juices. Raw carrots contain almost all of the minerals and vitamins needed by the human body. They are rich in vitamin A and good sources of vitamins B and C. Carrot juice may be taken daily.

Cucumber juice is rich in vitamin C.

Dandelion juice contains potassium, sodium, iron and vitamin A.

Lettuce juice is exceptionally high in vitamin A—more so than many other greens. It is also a good source of vitamin C. Among the minerals it is high in iron and magnesium.

Parsley is a very rich source of vitamin A, and also a good source of iron, sodium and sulphur. It's very strong and said to be a nerve stimulant. It will keep you awake like a strong cup of coffee.

Spinach juice has a high iron content and is very rich in vitamin A. Several ounces of spinach juice will give you enough for a whole day.

Watercress is another good source of vitamin A. It contains many minerals, particularly sulphur, and has a high iron content. It is alkaline because of its potassium content.

Try mixing carrot juice, celery juice and apple juice for a good basic drink. Double the amount of carrot juice to equal parts of celery and apple.

Each juice is rich in vitamins with the carrot offering vitamin A, the apple high in vitamin C, and the celery rich in sodium.

Or try an aperitif of tomato and apple juice. Tomato juice has a high vitamin A content and also contains vitamin C. It's a natural alkalizer and tends to neutralize the system.

Onions, radishes and pineapple blend into a juice that is nutritious and rich in sulphur.

Or put tender young beets through the juice extractor. Add grapefruit juice for a soothing alkaline drink.

Rhubarb and young asparagus mix well, with a touch of grapefruit to alkalize the rhubarb.

And tomato, celery and parsley make a juice rich in copper and iron.

With a little experimenting, imagination and taste will guide you in mixing your own varieties of health cocktails Or try those at your health food store for some far-out but nutritious combinations.

FAR-IN RECIPES

Health foods can be sensuous, spartan, exotic—anything your mood requires. To be nutritious is far from synonymous with being dull. A variety of naturally grown foods prepared with the gourmet's touch are presented in this section.

The recipes on pp. 149-153, 156-158, 160-161, 164-166 are reprinted with the kind permission of the publisher of *Adventures in Cooking with Health Foods* by Nancy Sutton, copyright 1969 by Nancy Sutton, published by Frederick Fell, Inc., 386 Park Ave. South, New York, New York 10016.

The recipes on pp. 154-155 are reprinted with the permission of the publisher of *The Soybean Cookbook* by Dorothea Van Gundy Jones, published by ARC Books, Inc., New York.

The recipes on pp. 159, 162-163, 167-168 are reprinted from *Eat, Drink and Be Healthy* by Agnes Toms, by permission of Devon-Adair Co.

Brazil Nut Chips make a delicious appetizer:

BRAZIL NUT CHIPS

1 lb. Brazil nuts (in shells)
2 tbsp. melted butter or oil
1/4 to 1/2 tsp. salt

To shell the nuts, cover them with water in a saucepan and bring to a boil. Simmer 5 minutes. Drain and shell. Cut into lengthwise slices about 1/8 inch thick. Spread on a baking tray, drizzle butter or oil over nuts, sprinkle with salt, stir around with a fork, and bake at 350° F for 10 minutes, stirring frequently with a fork to keep from burning. Cool. Makes 1 cup.

Try Peanut Sunflower Spread on bread or crackers, or as a filling for celery:

PEANUT SUNFLOWER SPREAD

1 cup old-fashioned peanut butter
(just peanuts and salt)
1/2 cup shelled raw sunflower seeds

Soften the peanut butter with a spoon and stir in the sunflower seeds.

For a cool, refreshing fruit cocktail, tangy and nutritious, you might want to serve Mixed Fruit Compote:

MIXED FRUIT COMPOTE

1/2 fresh pineapple
3 grapefruits
3 oranges
1 cup fresh, frozen, or canned peaches
   or apricots
3 bananas
2 ripe pears
One 10-oz. package frozen strawberries
   (slightly thawed), or
2 cups fresh strawberries
1 cup seedless grapes (optional)
1 cup sweet fresh cherries (optional)
1/4 cup Triple Sec liqueur
   (sweet wine may be substituted)

Mix together pineapple and the sectioned grapefruits and oranges with their juice. Add the peaches or apricots, sliced bananas, diced pears, strawberries, grapes (cut in half, if desired) and cherries. Pour liqueur or wine over the fruit. This may be served at once or refrigerated for a few minutes to let the flavors mellow. If it is going to be held in the refrigerator for more than a few minutes, wait until the last minute to add the diced pears and sliced bananas so they don't get mushy or brown. Other fruits, such as raspberries, blueberries, or melon balls, may be added. This fruit mixture may be served in scooped-out pineapple shells, cut lengthwise with foliage left on for a festive touch. Serves 8 to 10.

Salads can be exciting, nutritious and colorful. Use fresh, organically grown vegetables for this "Italian Slaw." The purple cabbage adds color, zest and vitamin C:

ITALIAN VEGETABLE SLAW

1 medium-sized head purple cabbage
1 medium onion, preferably red
6 stalks celery
1 green pepper
3 carrots
1 tsp. salt (preferably vegetable salt)
1/4 tsp. pepper (preferably freshly ground)
1/4 cup olive oil
1 to 2 tbsp. raw sugar
1/2 cup wine vinegar
1/2 to 1 cup mayonnaise

Shred the cabbage. Finely chop the onion, dice the celery and pepper, and finely grate the carrots. Mix all vegetables together. Combine remaining ingredients to make dressing and stir into vegetables. Serves 8.

Salads can also be simple, but exotic. Nancy Sutton's
Chinese Cucumbers are delicious and healthful:

CHINESE CUCUMBERS

> 1 large cucumber
> 2 tbsp. wine vinegar or cider vinegar
> 3 tbsp. soy sauce
> 1 tsp. chopped fresh ginger root
>   (available in Chinese grocery stores)
> or 1 small piece dried ginger root
> 1 tbsp. oil

Peel cucumber and thinly slice. Add remaining
ingredients and allow to marinate in refrigerator
for 1 to 2 hours or longer. Serves 4.

The soybean can be used in a variety of ways in salads. Dorothea Van Gundy Jones suggests a variety of ways in *The Soybean Cookbook*. Green beans and whole canned or cooked beans can be used in vegetable and molded salads; you can use soy sprouts either cooked or raw; and for recipes that call for nuts, try roasted soybeans.

Here's a delicious Soybean Vegetable Salad:

SOYBEAN VEGETABLE SALAD

1 can of 2 cups cooked soybeans
1 cup chopped celery
1 cup cooked carrots, diced or shoestring
1/2 cup diced cucumber
Watercress
Tomato slices

Drain beans, add celery, carrots, cucumber, and a small amount of watercress. Mix well, moisten with French dressing or soy mayonnaise, and place in lettuce-lined salad dish. Decorate with sliced tomatos. Serves 4 to 6.

For the additional nutritional value of the soy sprout, try the exotic Bean Sprout Sukiyaki:

BEAN SPROUT SUKIYAKI

2 cups vegetable protein food,
  shredded, or
soy cheese
2 tbsp. olive oil
2 tbsp. food yeast
1/2 cup green peppers, sliced thin
1 cup sliced celery
1 cup raw bean sprouts
1 large handful spinach
1 cup Chinese cabbage
1/2 cup green onions, cut into
  1-1/2 inch lengths
1 small can mushrooms
2 tbsp. soy sauce
1 tbsp. dark brown sugar or honey

Brown vegetable protein food in oil. Add food yeast, and then add the rest of the ingredients except for the spinach. Cover pan tightly, and cook mixture over low heat 12 to 15 minutes. About 3 to 5 minutes before serving, take off the lid and put in the spinach. Replace lid, and cook a few minutes longer. Serve with brown rice. Serves 6 to 8.
Sukiyaki may be cooked at the table in a chafing dish or electric frying pan, or it may be prepared over a barbeque pit. Serve in the container in which it is cooked.

Hopefully, the art of bread baking is being revived; the aroma and taste of freshly baked bread are worth the time.

If you would like to buy some fresh, stone-ground whole-grain flour from your organic merchants and bake your own bread, here are several recipes you might enjoy trying.

Nancy Sutton cautions that there are a few simple rules to follow, but it's quite easy to turn out delicious bread.

Yeast should be dissolved in warm water—not over 110°F for dry, granular yeast. If you use yeast cakes, have your water about 95°F. One yeast cake is equal to 1 package of dry yeast.

Whole-grain breads take longer to rise than white breads but don't allow your dough to overrise. And you should be aware that doughs made of 100 percent whole grains will never rise quite as high as those made with white flour.

Try delicious whole-wheat bread. It makes 4 small, nutritious loaves:

WHOLE-WHEAT BREAD

1 cup scalded milk
3 tbsp. molasses
3 tbsp. honey
2 tsp. salt
4 tbsp. oil
1 egg yolk
2 packages dry yeast
1 1/4 cups warm water
1 tsp. brown sugar

3 cups sifted unbleached white flour
1/2 cup wheat germ
1 tbsp. carob flour or powder
1 tbsp. soy flour
4 cups sifted whole wheat flour
1 egg white
2 tbsp. water

Scald milk. Place in a blender with the molasses, honey, salt, oil and egg yolk and blend a few seconds, or mix in a bowl with a mixer. Dissolve

the yeast in the warm water with the sugar for 5
minutes. When the milk mixture has cooled to
warm, add the yeast mixture. Add the sifted white
flour and the wheat germ and beat 1 minute with
an electric mixer. Sift the soy and carob flours
with the whole wheat flour and stir into the batter.
When well-blended, turn dough out on a floured
surface and knead 5 minutes, until smooth. Place
dough in an oiled bowl, turn greased side up, cover
with waxed paper and a tea towel, and let rise till
doubled (about 1 1/2 hours). Punch down and let
rise again till almost doubled (about 45 minutes).
Shape dough into 4 small, oval loaves. Set on oiled
baking sheets 3 inches apart and slash lengthwise.
Cover and let rise till doubled (about 45 minutes).
Beat the egg white and the 2 tbsp. water with a
rotary beater till frothy, and brush on the loaves.
Bake at 375° F for 20 to 30 minutes till done. Cool
on racks. Freezes well.
Note: This dough may be baked in two 9 1/2 by 5
1/2 by 3-inch loaf pans. Bake 10 minutes longer.

If you'd like to try some rye bread, Buttermilk Rye makes 2 loaves:

BUTTERMILK RYE BREAD

2 packages dry yeast
1/4 cup lukewarm water
2 cups buttermilk
2 tbsp. caraway seed
2/3 cup molasses (not blackstrap)
1 1/2 tsp. salt
1/4 cup oil
2 cups sifted unbleached white flour and
2 tbsp. wheat germ
2 cups unsifted whole wheat flour
2 cups unsifted whole rye flour

Dissolve yeast in lukewarm water. Let stand 5 minutes. Heat buttermilk till lukewarm. Pour into a large mixing bowl. Add the yeast, caraway seed, molasses, and salt. Beat in the white flour and the wheat germ. Add the oil. Beat well. Gradually add the rye and whole wheat flours to form a stiff dough. Knead 5 minutes, till smooth. Put into a greased bowl, turn greased side up, cover with a piece of waxed paper and a tea towel, set on an electric heating pad set at medium, and let rise till doubled (about 2 hours). Shape into two loaves and put into greased 9 by 5 by 3-inch bread pans. Let rise till doubled while covered in pans (about 1 hour). Bake at 325° F for about 40 minutes or till done. Turn out onto racks to cool immediately. Freezes well.
Note: This recipe may be made with sweet milk as well as buttermilk.

Agnes Toms, in her *Eat, Drink and Be Healthy* cookbook
has a delicious recipe for Oat Bread, using whole wheat flour,
soy flour and steel-cut oats:

OAT BREAD

6 cups whole wheat flour
1/2 cup soy flour
2 cups milk
1/4 cup oil
1/2 cup molasses
2 cups water
1 1/2 tbsp. salt
2 yeast cakes
1 cup steel-cut oats

Have all ingredients at room temperature. Sift
flour. Heat milk to lukewarm and add oil. Add
molasses, water and salt. Crumble yeast into
mixture and stir until dissolved. Add flour and
oats; knead 3 minutes. Allow to rise in warm place
for 2 hours. Shape into 3 or 4 loaves, place in
greased pans, cover with damp cloth and allow to
stand 1 hour. Bake at 375° F, 45 to 60 minutes.

Protein-rich menus can be planned around the more expensive cuts of meat or those that are less expensive but equally nutritious. Organ meats are high in food value; here is a tempting liver dish:

LIVER BOURGEOIS

1 lb. liver (any kind)
1/3 to 1/2 cup wheat germ
6 slices bacon
1 small minced onion
1 small minced green pepper
1/3 cup catsup
1 tsp. Worcestershire sauce
Salt and pepper

Slice liver into 1/2 inch slices and roll in wheat germ. Fry bacon till crisp. Drain on paper. Pour off all but 3 tbsp. drippings. Saute the minced onion and pepper in the bacon fat for 2 minutes. Add the liver and brown 5 minutes. Add the catsup and Worcestershire sauce and simmer until liver is done (about 1 minute). Add crumbled bacon and salt and pepper if needed. Serves 4.

Heart is one of the most nourishing meats:

HEART PATTIES

> 1 lb. beef heart
> 1 medium onion (optional)
> 1 tsp. salt
> 1/4 tsp. pepper
> Flour
> 3 tbsp. oil

Remove veins and fat from beef heart. Grind the heart in a meat grinder (or use your blender). Mix in the finely chopped onion, salt, and pepper. Roll the heart, made into 4 patties, in flour and saute in hot oil until done. Top with catsup. Serves 4.

Note: These may be baked in a moderate oven for 20 minutes instead of frying.

Agnes Toms' milk shake contains fresh fruit:

MILK SHAKE

> 1 cup fresh, cold milk
> 1/4 cup powdered milk
> 1 tsp. vanilla
> Crushed pineapple, berries
>   or other fruit
> Mashed banana, persimmon or dates
> Coconut powder, malted milk, or
>   nut butter
> Ice cream or sherbet
> 1 egg

Shake, beat or blend first three ingredients. Add those combinations from the rest of the list which appeal to your taste.

Carob will satisfy your chocolate cravings without the usual aftereffects:

HOT OR COLD CAROB MILK SHAKE

3 tbsp. carob powder
3 tbsp. powdered milk
2 tbsp. raw sugar or honey
2 cups milk
1/2 tsp. vanilla

Mix ingredients in blender until smooth. A pinch of salt may be added and the mixture heated, if desired. Serves 2.

Orange juice becomes protein punch when prepared in the following way:

ORANGE PICK-UP

2 eggs
1 cup fresh, cold milk
1/4 cup powdered milk
1/2 cup orange juice
Honey to taste

Beat eggs until thick and foamy; add milk and powdered milk; mix well. Beat in orange juice and add honey if mixture needs sweetening. Pour into tall glasses with ice cubes. Serves 2.

Nancy Sutton suggests Carob Syrup for use as a flavoring for milk or as a dessert sauce on ice cream:

CAROB SYRUP

1 cup carob powder
1 1/4 cups water
1/2 cup honey
1 tsp. vanilla extract

Stir water into the carob powder, adding it slowly and stirring well. Add honey. Bring to a boil. Boil 2 minutes, stirring constantly. Cool. Add vanilla. Refrigerate. Use 1 to 2 tbsp. syrup to flavor 8 oz. milk. Makes 1 1/2 cups.

Pumpkin Cookies are unusual, spicy and good to eat:

PUMPKIN COOKIES

*2 1/4 cups sifted unbleached white flour or
whole wheat flour
1/4 cup wheat germ
4 tsp. single action baking powder
1 1/4 tsp. salt
1 tsp. cinnamon
1/4 tsp. ginger
1/4 tsp. nutmeg
1/4 tsp. allspice
1/3 cup butter or margarine
1 1/2 cups brown sugar
3 eggs
1 cup mashed pumpkin
1/2 tsp. orange extract
1 cup chopped pecans
1 cup currants or chopped raisins*

Preheat oven to 400°F. Cream butter with sugar. Add the eggs, one at a time, and beat well. Sift dry ingredients. Add pumpkin, orange extract, and dry ingredients. Reserve 2 tbsp. each nuts and currants for topping. Add remaining pecans and currants. Drop by tablespoonfuls onto oiled baking sheets. Sprinkle the cookies with the mixed pecans and currants. Bake at 400°F for 12 to 15 minutes till lightly browned and firm. Cool on rack. Makes 3 dozen. Freezes well.

If you'd like to experiment with Halvah, the Turkish
candy made from the sesame seed, try this recipe:

HALVAH

1 cup ground sesame seeds
1/4 cup honey
A few drops of almond extract (optional)

Mix all ingredients together till consistency is
creamy but not sticky, adding more honey or
sesame seeds if necessary. Form into small balls by
rolling between your hands. Makes about 12
pieces. Store in refrigerator if kept for any length
of time.

There are delicious fruit and vegetable drinks which can be made to satisfy your taste and your imagination. From *Eat, Drink and Be Healthy* are some suggested combinations. Try those that appeal to you, and, as with all foods, experiment. There are many possible combinations to suit your taste.

If nuts or grains are to be used, they should be ground first, before the liquid is added.

Whole fruits and vegetables should be cut up before adding them to the blender.

These milk, fruit, and vegetable drinks make a nutritious adding to your diet.

To 1 1/2 cups liquid milk, soy milk, or yogurt, add 2 or 3 of the following:

> *1/2 cup orange, pineapple, or*
> > *berry juice*
>
> *1/4 cup frozen fruit*
> *1/2 cup skim milk powder*
> *1/4 cup dry whey*
> *A few almonds, pignolias, pecans,*
> > *peanuts*
>
> *1/4 cup fresh fruit or berries*
> *A few dates or raisins*
> *1 banana, cut up*
> *1 apple (peeled if sprayed), cored*
> > *and cut up*
>
> *1/4 cup carob powder*
> *1/4 cup powdered yeast*
> *Sunflower seeds*
> *1/4 cup molasses or honey*
> *1-2 eggs, separated, the white folded*
> > *in after the mixture has blended*

There are a variety of ways to serve yogurt:

SALADS

YOGURT SALAD DRESSING

Blend 1 cup cold yogurt with 1/2 cup chili sauce, 1/4 cup drained sweet relish, chopped parsley, and salt to taste. Serve as a dressing for tossed green or vegetable salad.

WITH MEAT

YOGURT MEAT SAUCE

Blend 1 cup yogurt with 1 can undiluted, heated tomato or mushroom soup. Season to taste with salt, herbs, and serve as sauce over meat loaf.

FOR DESSERT

YOGURT DESSERT

Sweeten yogurt with honey or brown sugar to taste and sprinkle cinnamon over top. Chill and serve.

Other Nash Quality Paperbacks Related to Health and Nutrition You'll Be Sure to Enjoy

THE MAGIC OF HONEY by Dorothy Perlman. The ancients appreciated the glorious taste of honey — symbol of love in story, music and poetry. Health-food enthusiasts have discovered, once again, honey's powers — its delicious flavor, medicinal qualities and natural nutritional values. Here is everything you'd like to know about honey: it's role in history, its wondrous energy- and health-giving attributes, its legendary possibilities as a fertility food and aphrodisiac. #8001 $1.95

ORGANIC MAKE-UP by Mary Gjerde. Whatever your age or skin type, nature provides an aid to protect and enhance your skin. Honey, eggs and milk; plant substances such as herbs, fruits, leaves and seeds; extracts and rich oils of almond, avocado and olive are all natural materials intended by nature for you to use on your skin and hair. And you will find all of these natural ingredients in your own kitchen at a fraction of the cost charged for their synthetic counterparts. #8003 $1.95

VITAMIN E: KEY TO SEXUAL SATISFACTION by Gary P. Brandner. Everyone's talking about Vitamin E. Here is a revealing account of how and why the amazing "E" has come to be known as "the sex vitamin." If a vitamin can be called topical, Vitamin E is just that. The author traces its history and documents how it heightens sexual capabilities and increases response and sensitivity during sexual encounters. #8000 $1.95

INTRODUCTION TO HEALTH FOODS by Marjorie Miller. This complete guide on how to prepare and enjoy health foods introduces the novice to the various types and forms of health foods, their nutritional value, the dangers of artificial preservatives, general principles of good nutrition, how to cook food so it doesn't lose its value, and exactly what foods are found in a health food store. #1187 $2.45

INTRODUCTION TO ORGANIC GARDENING by Chuck Pendergast. The author shows how organic gardening will improve the quality of the foods we eat and help restore the natural balance which has been destroyed by the use of pesticides and chemical fertilizers. Illustrates how to grow your own fruit and vegetables the safe, healthy and natural way. #1188 $2.45

Announcing
a New Solution to the Common Cold
by Dale Alexander:

The Common Cold and Common Sense

Vitamin C is only part of the answer, claims Dale Alexander in this revolutionary work dealing with the common cold. Author of the best seller, <u>Arthritis and Common Sense</u>, Dale Alexander presents a totally new understanding of the common cold, including nutritional secrets that he contends will not only help prevent your catching cold but will ensure your general good health.

This is a book on the common cold which fully recognizes the importance of sound nutrition in combatting the cold. The author introduces you to his original Common Cold-Preventive Cocktail — a new way of eating — which quickly helps to build resistance to the common cold, reduces the length of a cold, and in some instances aborts a cold within a day. He also offers a complete week of daily menus for those who are overweight, underweight and normal weight, which will further help build resistance to the common cold. His menus include recipes for the nourishing Alexander Vegetable and Fruit Salads.

Dale Alexander also offers observations from his years of study and research with doctors and common-cold victims. He contends that certain tempting foods and beverages are partially responsible for the common cold and points out the cold-causing danger of holiday and birthday parties.

If you follow Dale Alexander's sensible, pleasant, nutritional regimen and pay heed to what he claims causes the common cold, the author maintains that the results will be greatly desired good health — free of colds — and the ability to function on all fronts. #1172 $5.95

Now at your bookstore or order from Nash Publishing, 9255 Sunset Boulevard, Los Angeles, California 90069. Add 40c per book for shipping.

Sexual Power

Nutritional Approach

By Victor Gerardi

A noted expert analyzes the effect of nutrition on overall sexual performance . . . including new information on Vitamin E.

What effect does good nutrition have on the sex drive and sexual activity? Does Vitamin E really improve sexual performance? What about the other vitamins like A, B, C and F in relation to sex? What are the essential nutritional substances for efficient sexual performance? What are the consequences of undernutrition? Noted San Diego nutritionist Victor Gerardi discusses the importance of good nutrition to a healthy mind and body, and therefore to fulfilling and effective sexual relations.

He also discusses the effects of ancient aphrodisiacs, Oriental herbs, folklore remedies, a high protein diet, and the relationship of mineral compounds such as iodine, zinc, calcium, magnesium and potassium.   No. 1220 $5.95

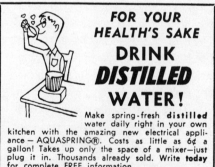
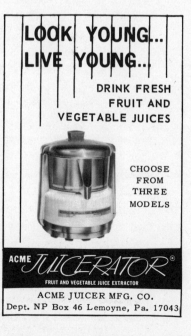

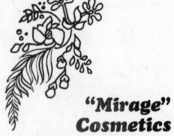

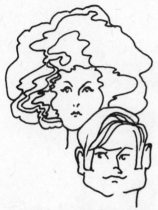
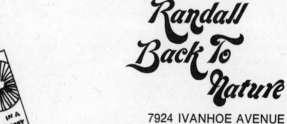
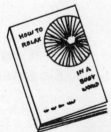